TO LOUISE

Angel of Light

R. Cook
Debbie Cook

Thanks

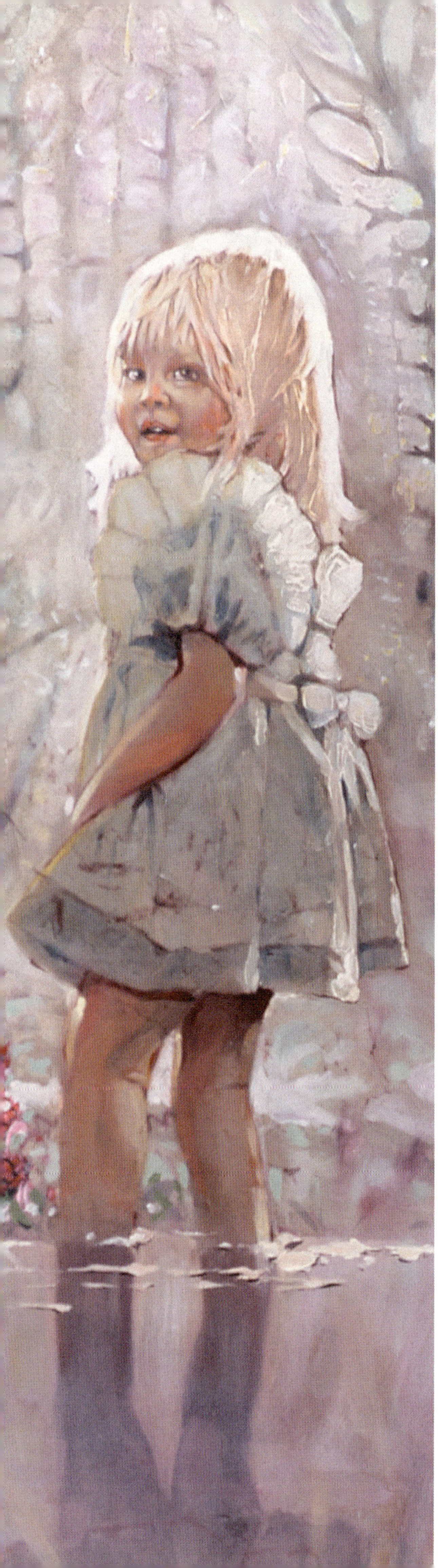

Angel of Light

A personal journey
through imagination
to find the spirit.

Written and with artwork by
RICHARD JAMES COOK

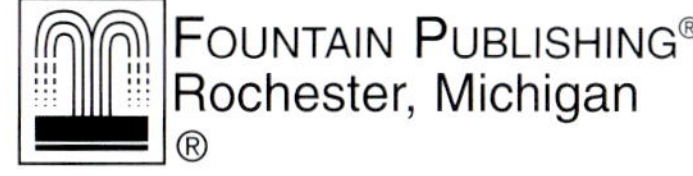

I wish to dedicate this book to Laura, our first child.
Without the experiences she brought into our lives,
this book would not exist.

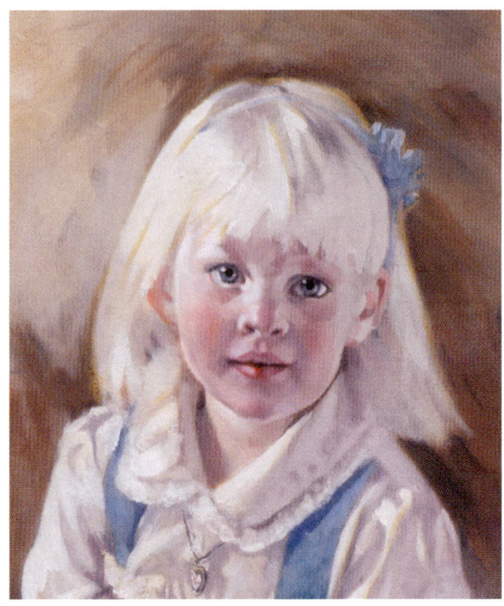

For thou hast delivered my soul from death,
mine eyes from tears,
and my feet from falling.

Psalm 116:8

Angel of Light

Copyright © 2001 by Richard James Cook
All rights reserved. No part of this book may be reproduced or transmitted in any form or by
any means, electronic or mechanical, including photocopying, recording, or by any information storage and retrieval system, without permission in writing from the publisher.

Published by Fountain Publishing®
P.O. Box 80011, Rochester, Michigan 48308-0011
www.fountainpublishing.com

Printed in the United States of America by McKay Press, Inc.
Book design by Richard J. Cook and 7th Generations Studios, Inc.

Library of Congress Cataloging-in-Publication Data

Cook, Richard James, 1955-
    Angel of light: a personal journey through imagination to find the spirit/written
    and with artwork by Richard James Cook.
        p.cm
    ISBN 0-9659164-4-8 (hardcover) ISBN 0-9659164-5-6 (paperback)
    1. Congenital heart disease in children. 2. Heart--Transplantation. 3. Spiritual life in
art. I.Title.

RJ426.C64 C66 2001
248.8'66'092--dc21   00-058704

Contents

Introduction

The grief following the death of one's own child is one of the most painful experiences a person can go through. Nothing can compare to having a little one, whom you would lay down your life to protect, pass away despite all your efforts.

Can anything good come from such a loss? Out of the depths of his pain after losing his four-year-old daughter, Laura, portrait artist Richard James Cook found a beauty flowing through his brush that he had never expressed before. Through the experience of being close to Laura's life and death, Richard discovered a new level of artwork - art that expressed the realm of the spirit.

"Angel of Light," the first of Richard's spiritual paintings after Laura's death, brought him a measure of reconciliation and comfort. Following this work, Richard went on to create many more paintings that depict more than just the physical eyes can see - paintings that reach into the realm where the spirit exists, where there is no death, and where God's presence is realized. He used these works of art as a means of exploring the reality where Laura now lives, and of finding a feeling of connection with that world.

The collection of artwork and poetry in this book is a gift to all those who want to receive it. Richard painted them not only for himself, but as tools for others to use, to find connections within the realities of spiritual beauty. His gift can raise our minds to the wonder of God, and the wonder of the eternal outpouring of love, comfort, and life that come from this one great Source.

The Story of Laura

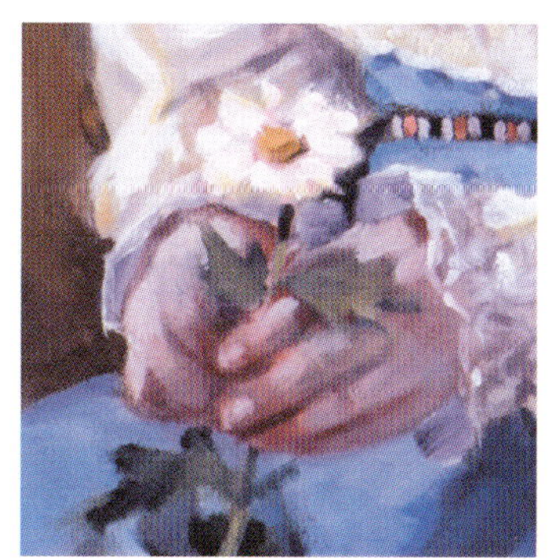

CHAPTER 1

A New Heart

My story begins on the 13th of September 1985, in a small delivery room at a hospital in Toronto, Ontario. I knew on arriving there that I was ill equipped to deal with what was to follow. Perhaps I should have been more attentive to those coaching techniques in the pre-natal classes. I have had little problem breathing for myself – I've been doing that for as long as I can remember – but I found I was not a natural at assisting my wife in her breathing as she entered into labor. Nevertheless, I managed to perform my role adequately, and my confidence was boosted by the confidence of the nurses, and by the feeling of being in good hands.

By 11:30 PM Debbie and I had in our hands our first baby, a girl. What a miraculous time that was. We had already narrowed down our choices of names for her to Laura and Elizabeth. We liked both names, and finally settled on Laura Elizabeth Cook.

It was the strangest thing, bringing this little bundle home to our small house in Etobicoke, Ontario. It was also one of the greatest experiences that I can remember. This homecoming marked the beginning of a number of adjustments for us – we found that babies need a lot of attention!

I think that it was during our Christmas visit with Debbie's family in Boston that we began to sense a problem. Laura was not thriving in a way that we felt was normal. A trip to the Hospital for Sick Children soon followed, and Laura was diagnosed with a rare heart disease called EFE or Endocardiofibroelastosis..

During the days and months that followed, we endured frequent hospitalizations and had to watch Laura struggle as cardiologists worked to balance drugs to support her weakened heart. Laura became our only focus. The cardiologists gave us statistics, and we learned that about a third of all children diagnosed with EFE fully recover from the disease, while a third of them remain the same, and a third deteriorate.

The best thing in our lives, Laura, and the worst, her illness, converged like two roads merging together. We were facing a new road, not knowing what lay ahead, and we felt helpless. The best that we could do might not be enough to alter the course that was shaping Laura's future. I am so grateful that God has been a central focus in our lives. I have found, with such focus, that the appearance of hopelessness can actually be the beginning of real hope. This is not the kind of hope that God would provide by the miracle of full physical recovery for Laura, although that would be nice. Instcad, this is the kind of hope that God's closeness would provide the strength to proceed on the difficult road ahead, and give us the vision to understand and read the signs, and to make the most of the sights along the way. It was not just Laura's destiny that was about to be shaped, but our own as well.

I cannot remember how early on it was suggested to us that a heart transplant was an option to consider in cases like Laura's. I can remember the thought sounding like something out of Aldous Huxley's "Brave New World." Yes, heart transplants were common in 1986, but they were still in a pioneering stage with young children, and were a last resort.

As time went on we did not see the signs of improvement in Laura's health that we had hoped for, and various infections would put her back in the hospital. One time when the fight against an infection was not going well, Debbie and I sat on the grass just outside Sick Children's Hospital having lunch, trying to make sense of the cardiologists' question: "If Laura goes into cardiac arrest, do you want her resuscitated?" How far we had come from that first day in the delivery room.

In spite of the tumult there was much for us to be thankful for. In many ways, Laura was a very normal child. Her favorite color was blue, and she loved to dance, just like many other little girls. But at the same time, Laura's strength showed her to be a most extraordinary child. Between her problem times she was usually very happy and inquisitive, and she loved people. I feel safe to say that those who came in contact with her were often touched in some special way. Her unique personality certainly was one of the sights along Debbie's and my shared journey that provided some of the strength we needed. Where did Laura find this strength and happy view of life?

I clearly remember the reaction she had when we brought our brand new baby, Ryan, home from the hospital. We were out in the back yard, and the day was bright and warm in early summer. Laura, just twenty-two months old, suddenly grasped the idea that this baby was ours, and was here to stay.

"Yes, Laura, he is your brother," we told her. She laughed and ran around and around the lawn chairs in unhindered happiness. We guessed that Laura liked the idea of a brother!

At the time of Ryan's birth and the months that followed, Laura did not have to be admitted back into the hospital, even though her heart function continued to deteriorate. In a strange way this was a reprieve. This became a special, bonding time for Laura and Ryan. They were inseparable, and grew to be the best of friends. We were all blessed by this window of health.

Before seriously considering a heart transplant for Laura, we went to Children's Hospital in London, Ontario, as they were the most advanced in pediatric transplants in Canada. Laura was three at this point, and her health was steadily growing worse. There we met with a team of cardiologist doctors who imbued us with more information about transplants than we could immediately understand. We were told that we did not have to make a decision right then, and could back out at any time. But with their estimation that Laura only had six months left on her present course, there was little choice but to put her on an active waiting list for a transplant. Yet another point had arrived on our road, one which involved new choices and the trained help of others.

Armed with a beeper, we were now on call twenty-four hours a day, living in both fear and hope that we would get a call. Three and a half weeks later we went to stay at the cottage of some close friends on the Muskoka lakes. The members of the Parker family were like family to us. Laura was very special to them, and she loved the cottage. The year before she had asked, "Can I come here next year?" This twisting of the Parkers around her little finger secured our visit to their cottage the following year.

At around seven o'clock Sunday evening, we had just finished packing to leave the Parker cottage after a wonderful weekend when the beeper sounded. A brief phone call informed us that a suitable donor heart had become available. We decided to leave little Ryan with the Parkers, which seemed a good idea to him, and began a race to get to London, Ontario. As far as the doctors in London were concerned, Muskoka, a three-and-a-half-hour drive away, was at the upper limit of acceptable distance. We had been fortunate not to be required to remain in London while a donor was sought.

A New Heart

For the first time ever, I ignored a long traffic jam and passed by on the shoulder, despite shouts of a few disgruntled on-lookers. If the police had stopped me, I probably would have gotten a much-needed escort. As I frantically drove, we explained to Laura, as best we could to a three-and-a-half-year-old, that she was going to get a new heart.

We arrived at the hospital in good time, only to wait and wait until finally, at one o'clock, Laura was wheeled through double doors and was gone. Debbie and I wondered if we would see her alive again. This was a six-hour surgery, so we had a long wait ahead of us. On his first visit from the operating room, the doctor informed us that the old heart had been removed, and they were getting ready to hook up the new one. I remember saying at the time, "I suppose it's too late to change our minds now?" Humor is a strange beast – it can show up at the oddest times, thank goodness.

Close to six hours had gone by when the surgeon, Dr. Menkis, informed us that all was still going well. The new heart had started to beat on its own as it warmed to body temperature, and he said that this was a good sign. For us, light began to shine in the tunnel. Tension was still there as the doctors finished the surgery, but the new heart, a great loss for some family in Denver, was pumping life into Laura – and wouldn't they feel some consolation if they knew her?

At nine in the morning it was over, and Laura was in intensive care and stable. For a brief time we were allowed to see her. There she was, hooked up to a ventilator, several IV lines and a drainage tube. Huge bandages were across her chest, but in spite of it all she actually looked better than she had in a long time. The mottled pattern that had marked her skin was gone, and she felt warm to the touch. It was encouraging to see her looking so well. She had made it through the surgery, and we would take one day at a time. But then, we had been doing that long before we considered a transplant.

One of the many blessings at this time was the opportunity of having a place to stay for the ten weeks post-transplant in London. The Ronald McDonald House provided a wonderful environment for families of children undergoing a transplant or chemotherapy. Ronald McDonald house in London was situated within the hospital complex. Spacious and well decorated, it was certainly our home away from home. It came with a common kitchen where all families staying there could prepare their own meals. This kitchen was also the room in which all would congregate, to share their incredible stories as to why they were there, or just to tell the day's events. We all felt like family sharing a common bond, for we each had our lives in the balance with a child either waiting for a transplant or recovering from one. Here, it was possible to feel close to a stranger in just a few days, and form friendships which in normal circumstances could have taken years. We all found strength through camaraderie. There would always be someone who was going through a more difficult time than you were, and you would be needed to offer friendship and support. We all took one day at a time.

After seeing Laura right after surgery, Debbie and I were only too happy to crash in our own room. A while later, we returned to intensive care and to Laura. On and off she was awake, and we could tell from her eyes that she was uncomfortable, asking, "Why did you let this happen to me?" It tore at our hearts that we couldn't make her distress go away.

In the Hospital

Day 2: Laura was staying awake now, and although there was a ventilator tube down her throat, she clearly mouthed, "I want a drink of water with lemon juice and ice." She was very upset that she wasn't allowed a drink, but she couldn't understand the doctor's concerns of lowering and monitoring the fluid build-up in her heart cavity. Early that afternoon, the ventilator was removed and she could talk. One of the first things she said was, "Get me out of here!" Two chest tubes were removed later that afternoon. Finally she was allowed a few ice chips which quenched her thirst for about two minutes! This was a good day even though she tired easily.

Day 3: The morphine and oxygen were discontinued. Although this left her more alert, Laura still slept most of the day. When she was awake, she wanted drinks, and fortunately more drinks were allowed now. It was a roller coaster of a day as doctors administered heart medication drugs to speed up her new heart. I remember watching those heart monitors racing at high speeds, and the doctors finally decided that Laura was too sensitive to the medications, and discontinued them. Although she couldn't communicate with us much, our presence was important to her.

There is a noticeable courage among the critically ill and their families. The bonds that Debbie and I made with other couples in that intensive care unit were immediate. The need to reach out was strong. You tend to forget your own needs when the needs of another outweigh your own. When we saw other parents who hadn't even had a chance to get to know their newborn before having to face these life-wrenching challenges, Debbie and I realized how blessed we were. We at least had been able to see Laura grow up a little first, and to laugh and to cry with her.

That day I had to leave for home in Toronto, and Debbie felt lost in my absence. Leaving was not easy for me either, but I had to be home for Ryan. We were not ready at this point to take a two-year-old into the mix of the London scene.

Back in intensive care in London, a sprite and friendly nine-year-old named Dallas was befriending Laura. Dallas had had a liver transplant right before Laura's transplant, on the very same day. Despite their age difference, nine-year-old Dallas and three-year-old Laura struck a kindred bond. Dallas and his parents were from Vernon, British Columbia. They were just one of the families who had travelled a long way to be a part of the pediatric program. Far from their own family and friends they reached out to others for support.

Day 4: Laura continued to progress well, but Dallas and his parents, David and Robin, had been given bad news. The latest test results showed that the transplant was not taking well, and that a second transplant would have to be done. This was devastating news, especially since, the day before, David and Robin had been told that Dallas was doing great! Such emotional swings, perhaps better described as roller coaster rides. But at least with a roller coaster you can see the end of the ride, and you have the choice of getting on it or not. We were aboard a very long ride with no visible end and no option to get off. What would the challenges be for Laura and for us in the days and months ahead? Would we be up against something big? If so, how severe? It's strange that despite all the trauma, it was the miraculous perseverance of the children that gave strength to the parents, even through the overwhelming reality that fate rested outside of our hands.

Day 5: Laura had an excellent day. She was able to have a full diet and ate well, better than she had in months. That day, she also gave out her first post-transplant smiles and laughs. She watched her favorite TV shows, "The Elephant Show" and "The Polka Dot Door," and must have watched the "Cinderella" movie thirty times! She had a keener interest in activities, and sat up for quite a while. Laura was back!

Day 6: I brought Ryan to London, and was very warmly welcomed by Debbie. Those two days apart had seemed so long! It was a real pleasure to be back, especially to see Laura sitting up and alert and just to be there with her.

This was a difficult day for Dallas. That morning he had his second transplant. The operation went well, and we attempted to be as supportive as we could to David and Robin. It was a tough day for them to be sure.

Day 7: I was eager to see Laura and, after enjoying coffee and a doughnut donated to the McDonald House by a local shop, I walked across the forecourt at around eight o'clock. It was a clear warm morning, and walking was a pleasure. My spirits were high at my home away from home. But barely minutes into my arrival at the hospital ICU, those spirits took a radical turn.

Laura was somewhat distant on my arrival. I noticed her legs twitching rhythmically, and I knew that this was an involuntary action – she was unaware that this was happening. I soon sensed that she was not visibly aware of anything. Then her eyes started twitching and rolling back, and I realized, with shock, that something was very wrong.

I wasted no time notifying the nurses, and qualified help surrounded Laura in a matter of seconds. She was injected with anti-convulsant drugs, returned to I.V. lines, and sedated. It seemed like an eternity, but was probably mere minutes – time and space do not exist in crisis. I noticed her body relax and the panic had gone – at least for now.

I grabbed the nearby phone and called Debbie, telling her to come right over. Was this to mark the final stages of our journey? This was too soon – we had come too far. Laura continued to have several more seizures and then ran into problems with her breathing. This was such a tense and frightening time.

The doctors incubated Laura to control her breathing. Doctor Menkis felt that the cause was possibly a reaction to the anti-rejection drug, cyclosporin. His greatest fear was that the cause could be due to a blood clot in her heart (a stroke), or bleeding in her brain; but an ultrasound and CAT scan did not show any internal clots or bleeding. Next the doctors needed samples of Laura's spinal fluid, and it was difficult to watch such samples being taken from this small, fragile child. Fortunately, all of the tests were negative, which just left reaction to the cyclosporin as the culprit. It was a relief to determine the source of the problem, even though cyclosporin was fundamental to Laura's survival. Doctor Menkis felt that Laura would be much better in the morning, but we would have to wait and see.

How frightened we were to have the tables turn so quickly! It helped to know that all of the parents, nurses and doctors in ICU were pulling for Laura. What a day!

Day 8: Laura was drowsy most of the day. A one-year-old baby on one side of her was bleeding heavily after surgery, and another girl was brought in from a horse accident in a coma. Two by two, each respective set of parents arrived in tears. The spheres on that day were far from ideal. The environment was taking its toll on Debbie, and I hoped desperately that tomorrow would be better.

Day 9: This was a much better day, so my prayers were answered. There was improvement. Gillian Parker came to visit, just what the doctor ordered, more as a tonic for Debbie than anyone else and a friendly shoulder to cry on. Regular visits from friends made it easier for me to return to Toronto for a couple of days. The short break from the hospital environment was good for Ryan and an opportunity to catch up on business. It was difficult to go, but any time I felt the need, it would be easy to jump in the car and make the two-hour drive to London.

Another patient whose progress came to be important to us was a young girl about the same age as Laura. Her name was Sandra. Sandra was having a rough time in the ICU. Her first liver transplant a year or so before was failing and she was in again for her second. The second surgery left her weak, and so she remained in ICU longer than most. Sandra had had her surgery two weeks before Laura. Her good and bad days went almost like clockwork, one day on, one day off. As Laura began her recovery, she immediately struck up a friendship with Sandra. Sandra's progress became important to her, and she would inquire often about how she was doing.

Day 10: Progress was good, and things looked even better when Dr. Menkis looked pleased. Tomorrow was to be a big day. Laura would finally get out of ICU, and move up onto a different floor in a private room. Dallas, too, would move to his own room. We felt sorrow for Sandra, who after a month in ICU was to watch two new friends be promoted to "Upstairs," only to be left behind at a time when she really needed them.

Day 11: It was frustrating to have to rely on phone calls to keep up to date with Laura's progress. Now I was returning to the hospital, and it would be a relief to see Laura and Debbie again. The last time I saw Laura, she had tired easily. I was looking forward to being able to spend more time with her, now that she was stronger. Today, I would get to see Laura on the 7th floor. She had moved to her own private room, which I heard thrilled her as much as the TV, the toys and the playdough.

As soon as I arrived I went straight over to see Laura.   When I entered, I was stunned. It could be that I was not expecting to see her sitting up, or it could be that I was surprised to see her happy and doing so well. It was all of these things and more. As I entered, Laura turned to me and said, "Hello, Daddy!" This may seem normal enough, but it stopped me in my tracks. The sheer love and innocence that we shared in that moment I will remember for all time. All I wanted to do was hug her and tell her how much I loved her.   Through all the past events that had brought me to this day with her, it was only then that I clearly saw how much a part of me Laura had become. To think that I could have lost all this so easily, so many times.

I spent a lot of time with Laura. It was fun to have her well to the point that we could really get some quality time. I did get a little over protective of Laura, but then a psychologist or any sane person probably would know why.

With Laura now in a private room we could become a family unit again. Ryan wanted to join in all of Laura's activities. This included lying on her bed and watching T.V., playing games, and even sharing Laura's meal tray.

Day 14: This was Laura's biopsy day. A tube would be fed from her leg through the vein to her heart for a sample of the heart wall. It is the only real way to assess that the new heart is doing well and not being rejected. Laura was heavily sedated for this, so when she woke up she was very groggy. She also had an ultrasound taken of her diaphragm. The ultrasound showed that her left side was not working, which accounted for her labored breathing. Often, a side product of the surgery results in damaged nerves. Fortunately, this corrects itself in time.

Almost a daily occurrence was a nurse arriving to do blood work. I certainly would cringe at someone putting a needle into my finger, yet Laura would take this in stride. After all, she would get a finger puppet and a sticker each time. After seeing a collection of about thirty, I marveled at the people who make all these woolen puppets, each one a little different.

Doctors continued to change the balance of Laura's medications, but by now she was adjusting to the mix and quantity.

Day 15: Time was beginning to drag, especially for Debbie who reminded me there were still two and a half months before going home. Laura continued to increase in activity and get stronger. We attributed her constant giggling to the drugs! She was walking a lot more, and was allowed to take short excursions outside. With a wheelchair we could pay short visits to McDonald House where Laura played happily on the toy car.

Laura painted a picture of our whole family complete with new heart and scar. It was good to see her positive about the whole experience now.

Day 16: Dr. Rosenberg made the suggestion of a weekend pass. To actually all go home for a couple of days! But this exciting prospect came with mixed feelings. We were concerned that Laura's blood pressure was still unpredictable, and this would not be monitored overnight if we were back in Toronto. We just didn't want it to be more a worry than a pleasure, so we didn't take advantage of this opportunity just yet.

As the days passed, Laura became more and more active, vibrant and lively. She was gaining weight, and genuinely becoming the person that we had only dreamed of - a child free from illness due to heart failure. Laura's personality blossomed. Her carefree nature and her love of others gave her a lot of attention. But still, some days she would be moody. Life in the hospital was an unnatural environment, and now that Ryan was living with Debbie, Laura became more possessive of her things. As the daily stresses took their toll on Debbie, a three-month minimum stay in London again looked very long indeed. The idea of a weekend pass began to look more appealing.

August 5th: Just over a month after surgery, Laura was having bouts of breathlessness. Doctors were concerned about the possibility of the heart being rejected, and they increased the steroids she was on. When Dr. Menkis arrived, he immediately decided that fluid around the heart was the source of the problem. In front of Laura's two squeamish parents he proceeded to drain this fluid, and even as it was being done she felt better. This process had to be repeated a few times. Laura also had periodic biopsies, to look for signs of rejection. One biopsy showed that there were signs of mild rejection. Despite being assured that most children at some point experience mild rejection, we were worried. Fluid around the heart and moodiness could have been signs of rejection, but fortunately an IV and a high dose of prednisone got things back on track.

August 14th: Debbie had a dream. She and Laura were home on an overnight pass when Laura died. Debbie screamed, called the ambulance and did CPR to no avail.

As August went by, Laura grew stronger, but the unnatural environment of hospital life took its toll on everyone involved. Debbie returned home to Toronto occasionally on weekends, and this provided some necessary familiarity of normal life. Just simple things, like going into the yard and checking out the vegetable garden, meant a lot then. Because Laura was now stable and doing well, being away for short periods was not so much of a worry. Laura did not find this easy, but I think she understood.

One time Laura was visiting McDonald House and she and I were watching a movie together - "Cinderella," of course. She was sitting on my lap. There was a part in the movie that showed a flight of stairs; they curved around and at the top there was an open door with blue light streaming out. Without turning, Laura said in a matter of fact way, "It looked just like that when I died yesterday." She always referred to the past by saying "Yesterday."

September 5th: This was to have been Laura's first day at school. That Saturday, with a day pass in hand, we all took a safari out of McDonald House on a day of adventure.

We headed towards Port Stanley on the shores of Lake Erie, where Laura surprised us by getting a lot more than her feet wet. Ryan also enjoyed the water. Families on the beach were amused by watching me chase a sea gull around on an errand of mercy. The gull required my services to free it from a fishing hook lodged in its nose and a line around its wing. It was the final dive-bombing on top of the bird that took away its freedom for enough time to dislodge the hook. The gull then flew off with not so much as a thank-you. We had fish and chips for lunch, reminiscent of life back in the Old Country, merry England, the country of my birth.

September 11th: It was tedious to all be staying in the London McDonald House now that required visits into the hospital were down to two hours a week. A visit with Dr. Menkis and Dr. Rosenberg launched the breaking news we were waiting for - if all went well, we would all be going home on Friday!

September 12th: Laura made a necklace for Sandra (still in intensive care) and insisted that Sandra's dad promise to deliver this to her today. Sandra's Dad seemed a little surprised at the insistence, but was happy to be the courier.

September 13th: It was Laura's birthday, and the whole world knew it. She was so excited, and did get many gifts. Laura had always gotten a lot of pleasure out of making things and then giving them away. Now family, friends and staff were returning her kindness.

News came later that day that Sandra had died. All knew that she was struggling, but were shocked by the news. A sadness fell over McDonald House, and the sadness hit close to home. It made us realize how vulnerable all the transplant families are. Laura asked a lot of questions about death, and wanted to know where Sandra would be going now. She wanted to know about heaven and what it was like there. She already instinctively knew that heaven was a pretty neat place, and was comforted to know that her friend was there.

CHAPTER 3

Home Again

September 14th: It was Friday, and for the first time since the transplant we could go home to Toronto as a complete family. Even though the exodus was only for a couple of days, it marked the beginning of a brave new start, and gave us exciting hope for the future.

From this time forward, our life approached normal again. By the second week in October we had been home together for a total of three weeks. Debbie commented on how delightful even the mundane activities were, like buying groceries for more than two days or going to the local stores. This newfound freedom did not let us escape the need to travel to London twice a week for tests; but the hospital visits gave us the opportunity to keep tabs on old friends like Dallas and his parents.

Laura continued to thrive. As a result of her anti-rejection drugs, she developed chipmunk cheeks and dark eyebrows. We protected her from groups of people, avoiding places like church or the mall, until the levels of drugs that suppressed her immune system could be lowered.

The fear of her heart being rejected always remained. Laura was getting a lot of headaches, which were a side effect of the anti-rejection drugs. When she caught a cold or got the least bit sick, we always feared that she might be going into rejection. For me, it was Laura's zest for life that provided the strength to be optimistic despite the unwritten future.

Eventually we were able to venture out more. This gave us more freedom, and gave Laura the opportunity to meet more people. Totally clear biopsies meant that we were down to one visit to London a week.

Laura now had a different personality than the one we remembered from before the transplant. She had always been talkative, but now she was also active and stimulated. Instead of always sitting and watching at play school, she would often initiate activity. She had been given a new freedom to develop mentally and grow in a normal manner, and developed quickly in a short amount of time.

There was some cost to this growth and normality – Laura lost a little of her former innocence, and would now stamp her feet or find a room to pout in if things didn't go her way. Her mood swings were not all her fault. The medications played some role in the way she felt.

Laura was now a complete person, and not the delicate shell we once knew. The mischief I sometimes saw in her eyes told me that Laura was not yet an angel, and was firmly rooted on this earth. This, in a strange way, was a comfort.

November 1989: Laura was very excited at being asked to be a flower girl in a friend's wedding. She took the role most seriously, and the event went without a hitch. It wasn't until we saw some of the photographs that I realized how short Laura was, standing there with her bouquet and everyone else towering above her. She still had some catching up to do.

December 1989: We all had a lot to be thankful for as the Christmas season rolled around. It was a busy time for Laura, threading beads and making delicate envelopes to put the necklaces in. These would be distributed to close friends.

January 20th 1990: Debbie took Laura to London for a check-up. At this point visits were only once a month. Laura had done very well since her last visit, except for one day in which she came home from school and said, "It feels like my heart is leaking." It was good to be able to ask Dr. Rosenberg about this event, and he felt that it could possibly have been a heart rhythm irregularity. If it happened again, Laura would need to get a portable monitor to assess the problem.

January 24th: It was a big day for Laura, and she was especially excited. The class was going to the aquarium and then to a birthday party for two of her friends at McDonald's – the restaurant! Laura had spent a long time the night before decorating presents with stickers and drawings. She was so happy, sure that her friends would love the presents.

The temperature was cold that morning. As I drove Laura to school, the sun low in the sky played tricks with my eyes. I took a left turn onto the street that our church school was on. The unfortunate result was a head-to-head collision with another car. It was difficult to decide what to focus on. Laura had bumped her head and was crying, so instinctively I decided to leave the scene and get her home. After she was safely with Debbie, I went back. A policeman scolded me, saying that I shouldn't have left the scene. I was confused, my mind shifting from his reprimand to thoughts of Laura. I wondered how she was doing. The car had to be fixed, and fortunately a friend loaned us another in the meantime.

When I got home after all this, Laura was a lot better, except for a headache. By 10:00 AM she really perked up, and this time I let Debbie take her to school. She had a wonderful day and didn't return until 3:00 PM after the party. She was so full of excitement, and we were told by those running the party that they were amazed how energetic and active she was, and how much fun she was having.

That night, Debbie snuggled with Laura in bed and said prayers. After prayers Laura sat up in bed and said "Mommy, you know, I love you so much," and gave her a big hug.

January 25th: Laura woke up and climbed into our bed. Debbie then had to get up, but Laura stayed there in bed to snuggle with me a bit longer. She always loved her snuggles, but this was an especially treasured moment. I can't remember what we talked about, but I do remember as if it were yesterday when she said to me, "Do you know what, daddy? I love you."

Soon Laura got up to get ready for school, and had breakfast. Debbie and Laura then left on the ten-minute walk to the church school. On the way, Laura told Debbie how much she loved school and being with her friends. Her best friend was Janine, who had been born in the same hospital as Laura on the same day.

The sun was at 45 degrees, and shone down brilliantly through the soft wintry clouds like a halo of light. Laura looked up at this sight and said, "Mommy, it is such a beautiful day." Then she said, "See the sun? That's like the Lord in heaven." A marvelous concept from a four-year-old. Is that how the angels see the Lord in heaven?

Each morning at Laura's church school began with a short worship service. On this particular morning, Laura got to perform the job of opening the Word. After doing so, she turned to tell her friend and teacher, Gillian Parker, "That's my favorite job." During the worship Gillian reminded Laura to close her eyes when saying the Lord's prayer. Laura had a habit of keeping her eyes open, and, true to character, she asked why. Rachel, another girl in Laura's class, told her, "Because you can see the angels better." To this Laura replied, "But I can see the angels with my eyes open!"

When recess came Laura went out to play with some of the older children. A teacher recalled hearing her laughing with delight. Her laugh was distinctive to her teachers, and she used it often.

As recess came to a close, Laura came in with the other children. After coming down the stairs, she complained that her chest hurt. Gillian sensed that this could be trouble. As a trained nurse, she felt that getting Laura home immediately would be better than anything she could do there at school.

I took the call from Gillian saying that Laura was on her way home, sick with chest pains. Our friends Phil and Amy were driving her home. When I heard about Laura's problem, a chill went through me. Debbie had gone out, but by luck she arrived home just seconds after the phone call. She had come back to get her wallet for grocery shopping. I ran out to her and said, "I'm so glad you're here! Laura's sick." While I explained Gillian's call to Debbie, Phil and Amy arrived with Laura. Phil carried her into the house and she looked very ill. She had already been sick in the car, and when she came in the house she was sick some more. Debbie took care of Laura while I called Dr. Rosenberg, but I couldn't reach him, so I called Dr. Mansen, our local pediatrician. Dr. Mansen told us to bring her in right away.

Laura was crying out that it hurt, and was also a little delirious. She couldn't really stand, and was covered with a cold sweat. We were very frightened by now. We were both fearing "rejection," and did not know where all this was going. It was terrible to see Laura in so much distress and be powerless to make it go away. We quickly stripped off her clothes and put her into pajamas, as these were the easiest to put on. Should we have gotten an ambulance? In the panic we did not even think of it.

When we arrived at the doctor's office, we had to wait a short time. It would have been understandable for us to have rushed in to the office under the circumstances, but we waited anyway.

When we were finally called in, Laura was afraid to have the doctor touch her. After examining her, Dr. Mansen said that her heartbeat was very weak, and he called 911 to dispatch an ambulance. When asked about her condition, he answered, "She looks pretty bad." During this phone conversation Laura was sitting on Debbie's lap. Debbie and I were frightened, trying to do whatever we could to help her. Suddenly Laura went very pale. Her head fell backwards, her eyes rolled upwards, and then they closed. Terrified, Debbie said to the doctor, "I don't think that she's breathing!" The doctor quickly finished the call, listened to her and started CPR right away. Debbie assisted the doctor by breathing into Laura while he administered the heart massage.

As if time stood still I stared at Laura. I don't know if it physically happened, but after her eyes closed I saw them open again. They were focused and so peaceful.   I remember wishing I could see what she was seeing. Wherever it was that she was going, part of me wanted to go there, too. I shook with the power that I was sensing. It was as if two giant loving hands had come down to carefully scoop Laura up. I knew then that she was gone.

Twice Laura started briefly to breathe on her own. Everything was happening so quickly, and I rushed downstairs to wave down the ambulance. It seemed an eternity until it arrived, though it really wasn't. I led the medics to the second floor, to the room where Laura still lay, receiving the efforts of CPR. In my mind somewhere there had been a small hope that she would be sitting up.

I remember looking at Debbie and saying, "I think that this is it." It was a strange and chilling moment, and really the only moment since the morning phone call from Gillian that we had had time to stop and evaluate what was going on.

 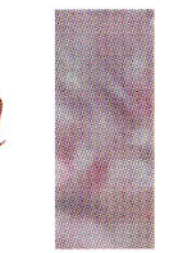

Once there, the medics took over and somehow managed to get Laura onto a stretcher without interrupting CPR, although they did stop while they took her down the stairs. In all of this we forgot about Ryan, who was hanging onto Debbie's leg. I wonder what was going through his mind?

It was decided that Debbie and Dr. Mansen would go in the ambulance to the hospital. There was room for only two plus the medics.   I stayed behind to try and reach Dr. Rosenberg in London. Luckily, the time between paging him and talking to him was short. I told him, "Laura's on the way to the hospital, she's on CPR and they are trying to resuscitate her. She started breathing briefly a couple of times – what should we do?"

There was only silence after I stopped talking. Then Dr. Rosenburg's slow, trembling voice replied, "She's gone into rejection; there is nothing to be done. Give me the name of the hospital. I will talk to them there."

I left Dr. Mansen's office to find someone to look after Ryan. I went to our church and would have just left him with Gillian who, although in the middle of teaching, would have been happy to help. Fortunately, I saw Rachel (a friend) as I drove into the church parking lot. I don't think I even got out of the car when I said, "It's Laura, take him," and left.

I made my way to Lake Shore Boulevard by Lake Ontario and on to St. Joseph's hospital, halfway between the doctor's office and downtown. I had to stop for gas (of all things) and in the panic had left without my wallet. The last thing I wanted at a time like this was to run out of gas. I stopped at a gas station, and the attendant must have read the urgency in my face when I said that I had no wallet. He said for me to take ten dollar's worth and pay him back some other time. Back on the Boulevard, there were road works and an officer directing traffic. I slowed down and asked if I were close to the hospital. He told me, "Yes, it's just over there, a mile on the left, can't miss it. You hurry now, and be careful." How do these people know what's on my mind?

Leaving the car at the front entrance of the hospital, hoping my friend's car wouldn't get towed, I ran in the main emergency entrance. The first person I saw, from some distance, was a nun who looked to be in her late sixties. She was looking at me, and started to approach. I knew it was all over. I cannot remember what it was that she said, but I do remember the heavenly sphere that surrounded her as she took my hands. There was comfort. She led me to the room where the doctors were still attempting to resuscitate Laura. They were waiting for my arrival, so that Debbie and I could make the decision to stop their efforts, which we did. The room was cleared, and we said our good-byes to dear Laura alone.

It was the strangest moment. Neither of us was crying. It was as if this were too tender a moment to waste on tears. Gillian arrived, and expressed all the emotions we were feeling. It was so right to have her, one of Laura's and our closest friends, share this time with us.

Yes, it was true that Laura's journey on earth and ours with her had come to an end. It was also true that this ending marked the beginning of an incredible new journey for her. Laura had shown a love for life. In her way, she had said goodbye in telling us how she loved us, seeing the Lord as being like the sun, and seeing the angels with her eyes open.   There was peace. Laura had been touched by the Lord, and through her innocence so had we. Grieving, I sensed, was not to happen today. Debbie and I made the best of things, as tomorrow would mark the beginning of our struggle on the long road toard healing.

CHAPTER 4

Connections

I cannot believe that it has been ten years since the day that we said goodbye to Laura. So much has refilled and changed our lives since then. It must also be true that Laura's life in her new world has seen many changes and challenges.

I had a dream days after she died. I was in a park; the grass was very green and the sun shone brightly. Laura was some distance in front of me, facing me. I was overcome with regret and loss. She smiled, and with lips closed told me, "It's all right." Then we were walking hand in hand, enjoying each other's company and the beautiful day.

The changes that Laura's absence caused in our family were immeasurable. Ryan was two and a half when she died. He and Laura had been exclusive play-mates ever since he was born. Ryan missed Laura terribly, and to this day, on some level, he still longs for his older sister.

Certainly the birth of Daniel two years after her death marked the "New Beginning" for us. For me, his birth rekindled a closeness; a kind of bridge to some of the lost affections that Laura had spirited. Laura must have been excited when Daniel was conceived. In spirit, she probably knew long before we did that Daniel was on the way.

Daniel reminded me much of Laura, and it was a treat to watch his personality grow. Daniel also shared something else with her – a link that rekindled old fears. He was diagnosed with a mild form of the same illness that Laura had. Fortunately, as the years went by the evidence of the disease decreased.

Laura continues to be an important member of our family. Our two younger boys, Daniel and Joshua, have a strong love for Laura even though neither has met her. They both love to go through all the family photo albums over and over again. They talk about Laura as if they know her. When Debbie's father died last year, Joshua said, "Oh, Laura will be there to greet him." Joshua is now six years old.

It has become more and more apparent to me that there is a hidden thread that constantly connects the Lord with us. There are connections through our daily existence to be perceived and interpreted. These connections not only open up our relationship with people here, but also with heaven and the Lord. In my case, these connections have led me and have pointed the way in which I should go.

Are our lives here on earth a preparation for life or a preparation for death? The answer is yes. Although I did not see the connections between events at the time, they have become apparent to me now.

Was Sandra's death and Laura's insistence to know exactly where she had gone a preparation for accepting heaven as a good place to be? I feel certain that it was. At the Christmas tableaux, three months after Sandra's death, Laura wanted to know if Sandra was on the stage with baby Jesus. To her, the scene was not just a representation, but real.

What had Laura experienced when she "died yesterday," as she informed me while we watched the Cinderella movie at McDonald House? Life is a series of preparations, and so, it seems, is death. And in His mercy, the Lord prepares us for great crossroads in our lives, as He did with the special moments Laura shared with us on the day of her death.

There is a reason for all things. Laura's life and death were not a result of random chance. I know almost nothing about astrology, but I do believe that the connections of the alignments of the sun, moon and stars do bear relation to spiritual events. Was it by more than chance that Laura was born in September on Friday the thirteenth on the birth of the new moon? Perhaps the ancient wise men who saw a bright star in the east could have told me that.

Was it by more than chance that just a few weeks after Laura's death I was compelled to paint a picture of her resurrection, which I've called "Angel of Light"? This painting helped me find reconciliation and comfort.

"Angel of Light" then went on to make other connections. Dan, a minister in our church and good friend, has led backpacking expeditions for years. In fact, Debbie had gone on two trips with him in Wyoming before she and I met. In 1989, back before Laura's death, Dan and his son Danny were out on one of these trips when tragically Danny slipped and fell on some rocks, hitting his head. Danny's condition was very serious, and he and his companions were miles from civilization. Dan and two others climbed out of the canyon at night to find help, and in the early morning Danny was airlifted to the nearest hospital. There, it was determined that his brain stem was broken, and he would soon die. Dan and his family were asked if they would be willing to donate his organs for transplant. Thrust into the finality of no hope for recovery, they believed that hope could be restored, if not for themselves, perhaps for someone else. Danny's heart gave life to a father in Utah.

Danny died on August 13th 1989. At that time Laura had been growing strong for six weeks on a donated heart. When we expressed our sorrow to Dan and his wife, Ruth, it in some way comforted them that Laura was alive by an anonymous heart donor in Denver – to see loss and gain as two sides to a coin. Later, when I showed them "Angel of Light," they were especially moved by the image and by the words I had written to go with it. The painting made a connection in their lives. They could imagine that Danny and Laura were perhaps becoming friends in a way that was similar to the development of Laura and Dallas' friendship – through shared circumstance. Imagination can be the gateway to perception I believe, provided that the Lord is in it.

Was it by more than chance that one evening I saw the northern lights for the first time (and the last so far)? In itself perhaps not. But minutes before, I had been telling Debbie that I really believed the Lord wanted me to make time to paint things that have spiritual importance to myself and others. "Angel of Light" had shown me how. I then went out in the car and saw a brilliant display of the northern lights. It seemed to be a sign of confirmation, that yes, this path was the one to follow. I thought of turning back to show Debbie, but something told me that the display was for my eyes only. I watched them for five minutes, and then they were gone.

I have presented these paintings numerous times and have been amazed at how people have been moved in different ways. "Angel of Light" was in an exhibit one year, and a woman whom I didn't know came up to me, threw her arms around me and said, "Thank you." She had recently lost a child, and the painting had made a connection for her. She said that now she could see what heaven was like for her child.

Connections

A word should also be said about the publishers of this book. After a presentation of these paintings at a convention called "Little Angels" in Bryn Athyn, Pennsylvania, I was approached to do a painting for a certain lady of her granddaughter. The granddaughter's name was Annica. Annica had died as a result of a tragic car accident. This woman, her grandmother, wanted me to paint her as she might appear in heaven. With pictures of Annica and some wonderful drawings she had made I was able to make a painting, which I have called "The Stars, the Dove, and the Secret Garden." Annica was the daughter of Jon and Karin Childs, who are the publishers of this book.

Ten years after redefining Laura in my life, I am writing a book dedicated to her and her connection with my life. It is amazing to me that, as I got to the point when I first wrote down the moment of Laura's death, it had been ten years to the day since she had died. I looked at the time and I asked Debbie, "She died around 1:00 PM, right?" The time on the clock was 1:00 PM. Ten years ago Laura said in a dream, "It's all right." I believe that she was right.

This book is a testament to the way the Lord's path shapes one's destiny. The paintings here shown are not just for me, although I enjoyed painting them. For me, they are tools whereby I can explore in imagination a means to find a connection to spiritual closeness. This closeness is unlimited and universal to all. The paintings are about issues that we all can identify with in some way, and are a means to that end. Some of them are commissions from others looking for inspiration, and others are where my own imagination has taken me. I hope that in some way this book reaches deep into the lives of others, bringing peace of spirit, in the same way that these paintings have brought peace to my life.

The Paintings

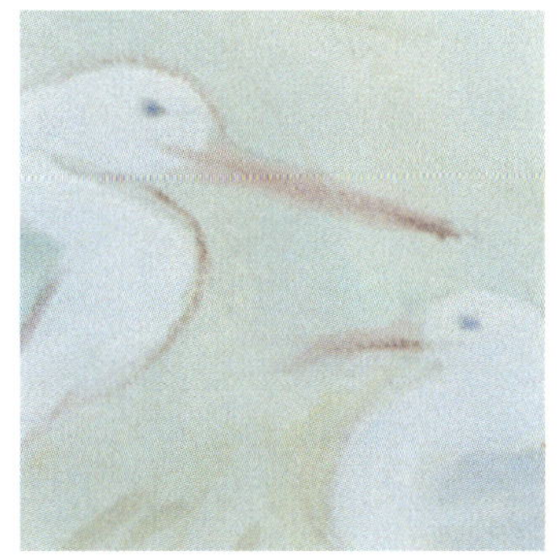

This painting was the first of its kind. "Angel of Light" was created a few weeks after Laura died, and it was the first time that I was able to use my skill as a painter to express spirituality.

While painting, I felt that it was not my hand that was guiding the brush. I was there merely to paint, to listen and to learn. Through the experience I found hope and reconciliation. Peace exists in the imagery and the movement of the paint.

With the completion of this painting, I believe the Lord had shown me a door and an opportunity. In this way, I can express an awe of the spirit through my art.

Angel of Light

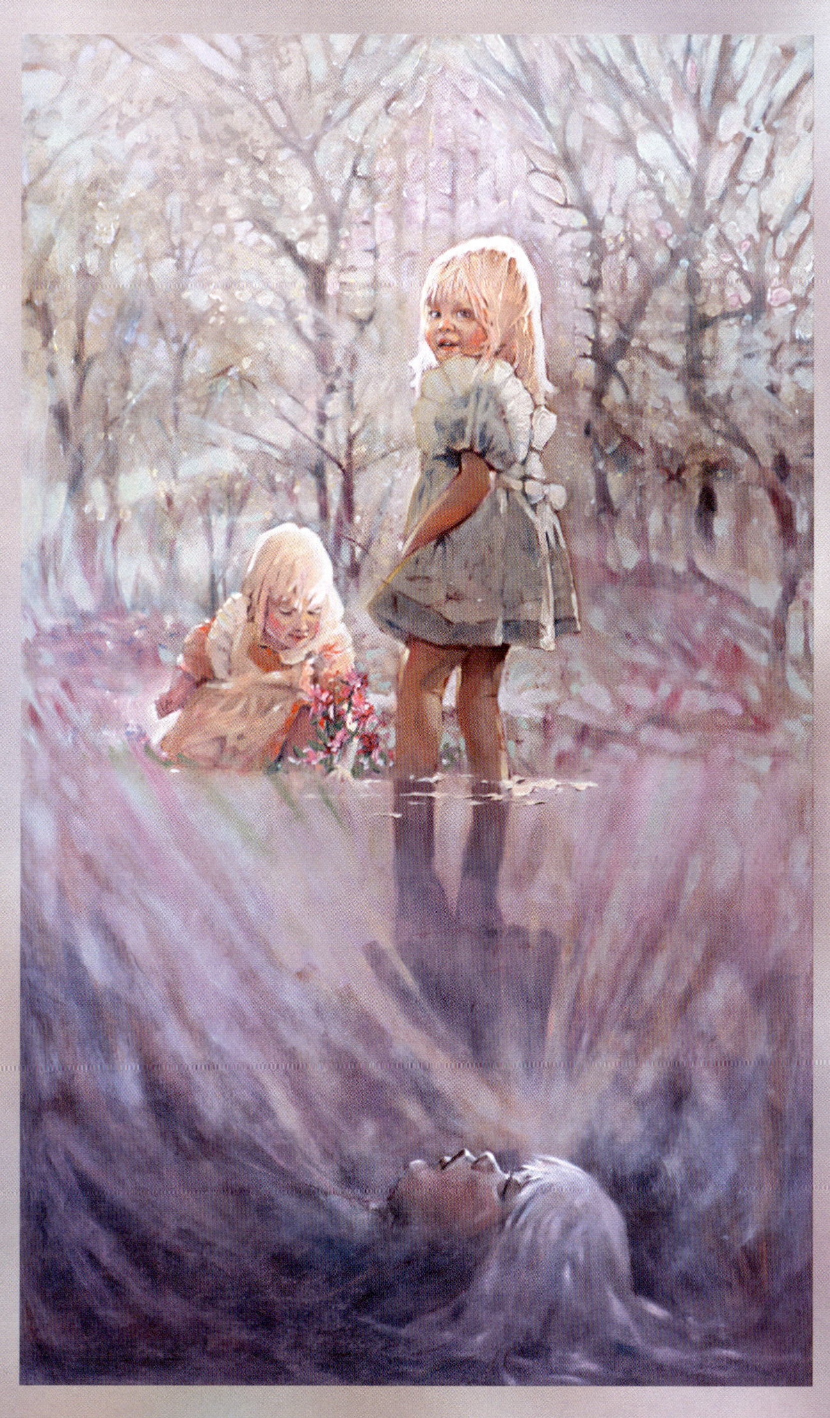

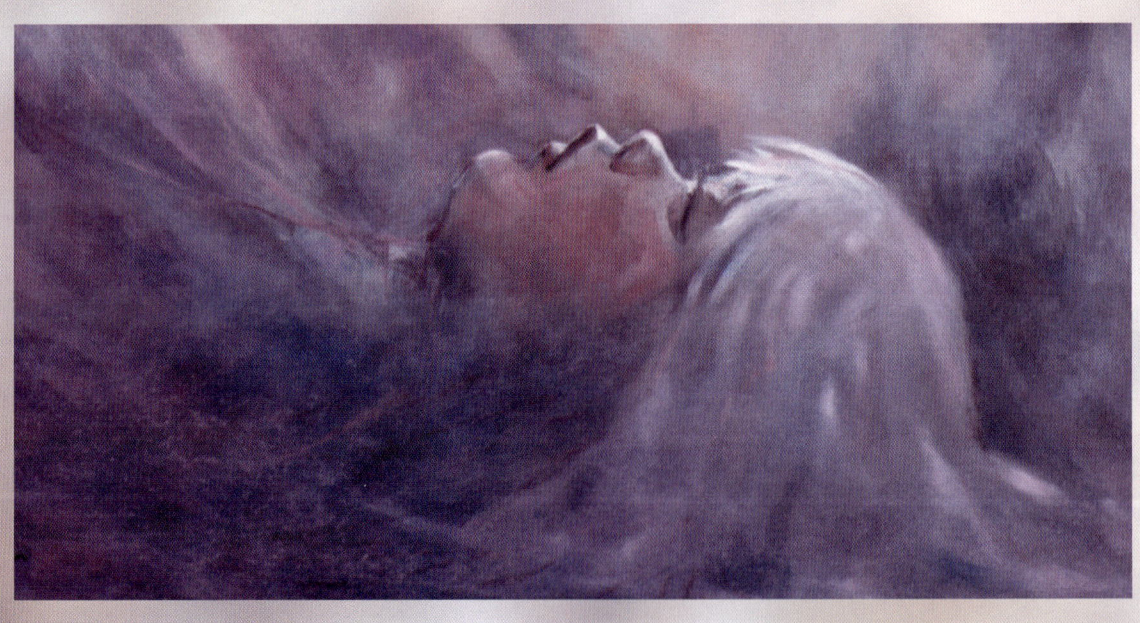

Our minds are persuaded toward doubt. Death is irretrievable –
why this pain? Was this love all in vain?

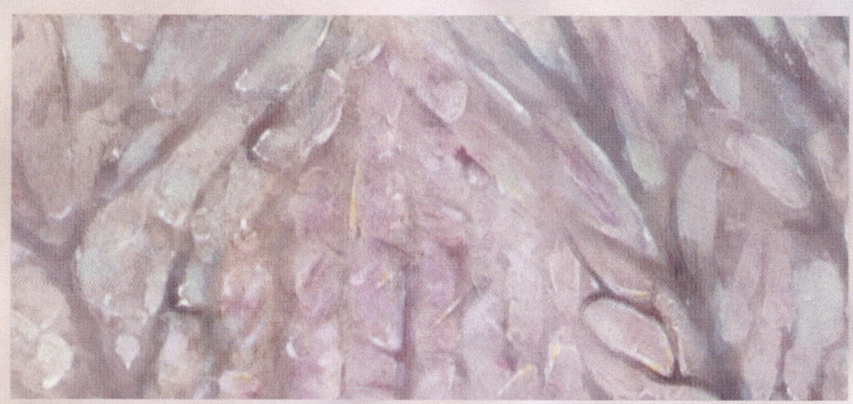

There is a deeper persuasion from within.
There is much more. The peace of death pays witness
to the wonders of creation itself, to the powerful hand of God,
ever uplifting and renewing.

She is but asleep,
only to be lifted to a new day.

Where is she now?

Where she always was – within us, as our love is within.

More, the kingdom of the Lord lies within us.

Where the Lord is, she is also.

Her joy and peace speak inside us, if we do but listen.

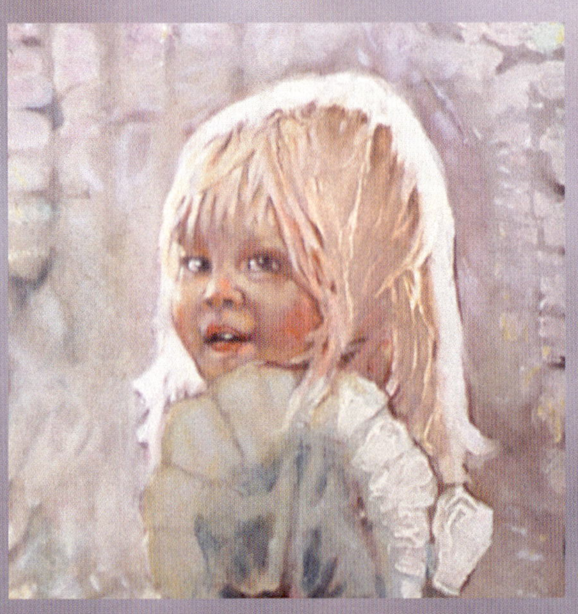

Hers is the beginning of an incredible journey.

She shows the way, almost beckoning.

The water is good to the touch.

Her innocence makes it look easy.

A glance back admits excitement for the future,

but sadness in parting.

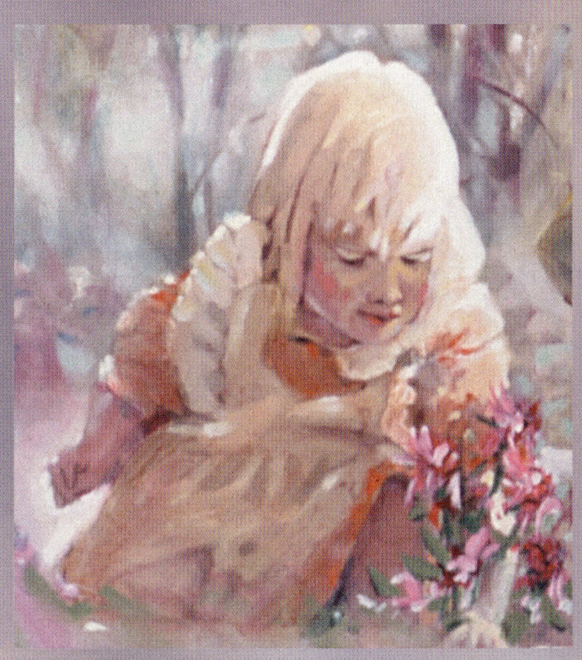

How I wish ours was a place
without time or space.
The pain of grief and parting,
for her, is brief.

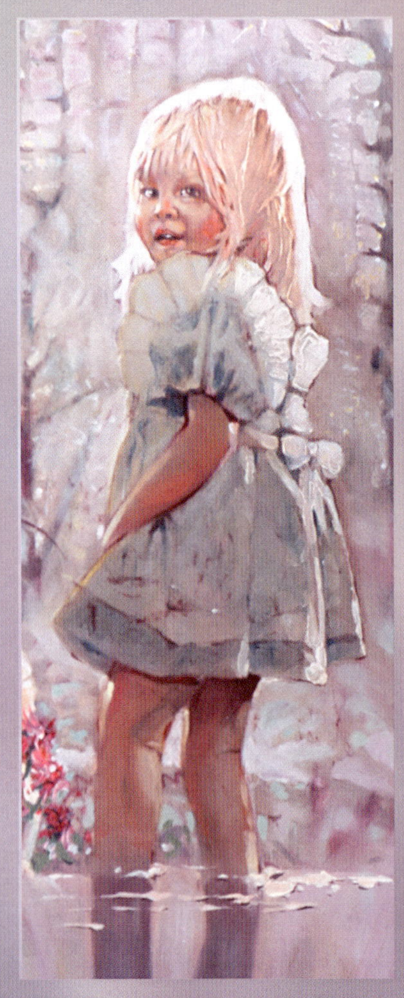

Her shadowed reflection in the water
whispers a bridge that spans the divide.
Past experiences and memories
will bridge both worlds,
until we too are on that side.

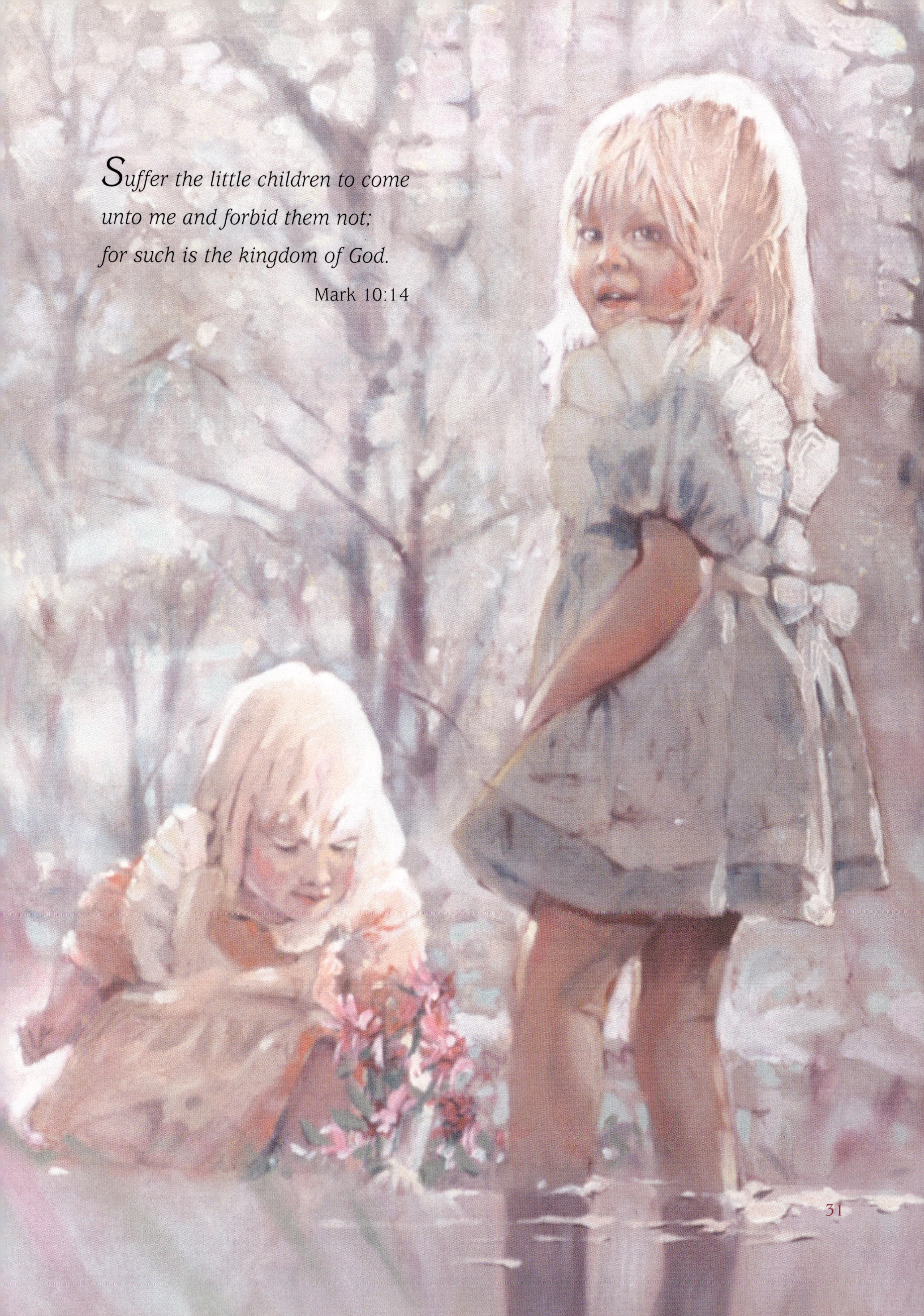

Suffer the little children to come
unto me and forbid them not;
for such is the kingdom of God.

Mark 10:14

This next painting was inspired by my wife. She wanted me to create a painting that might give an insight as to where Laura was, and what she might want to share with us now, two years after she had crossed into the spirit.

Before Daniel was born, Debbie and I speculated that perhaps Laura would somehow know the baby before we did – would see him before we did.

When I was working on this painting, Daniel was a year old. Once again I wondered if Laura had seen Daniel. It was just one of those crazy notions. I brought Daniel into my studio, held him in front of the painting and waited. If ever there was a time for one of those signs, here it was.

Daniel looked at the painting and said, "Raura." Then he turned to me, looked into my eyes, and kissed me.

The Eternal Dance

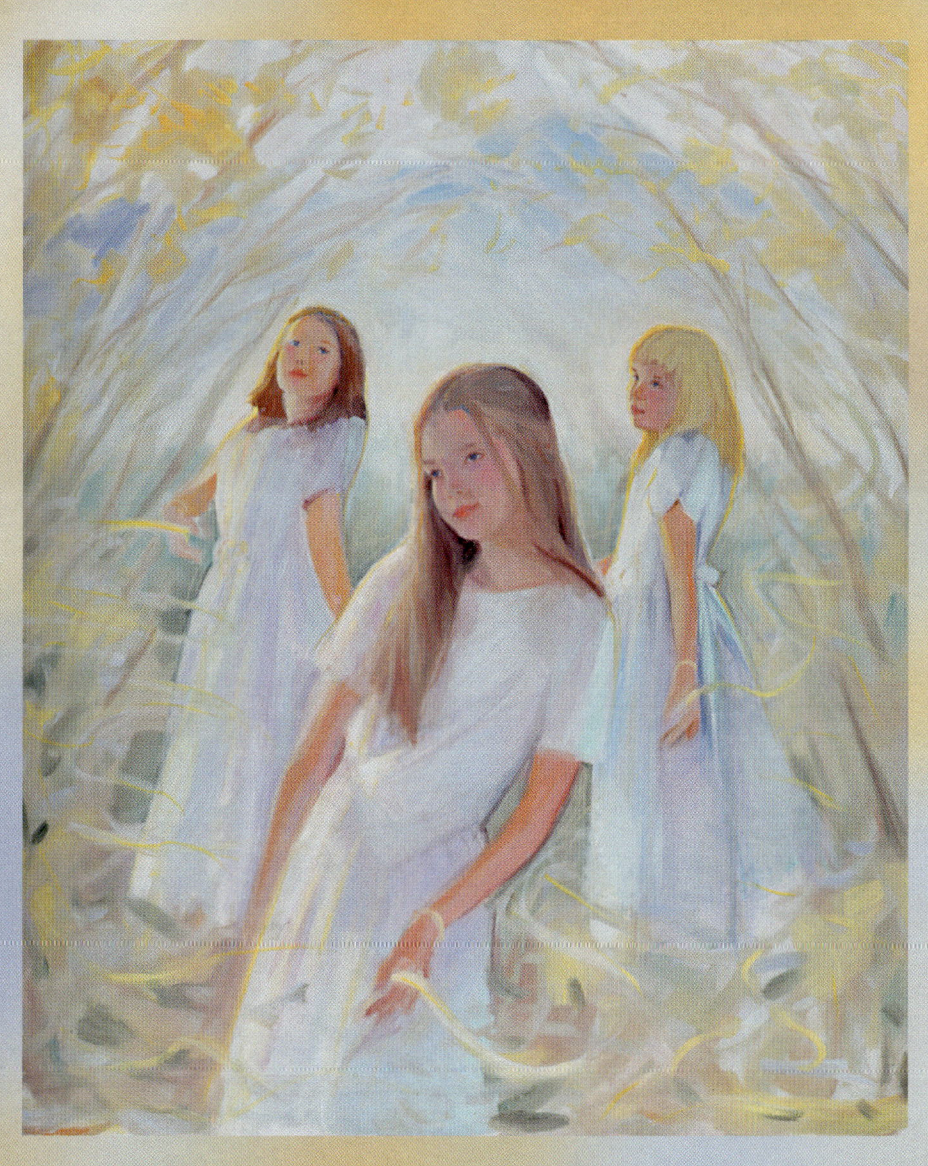

Is my memory fading? No, it serves me well.

Was it the laughter, the gifts you gave,

or the stories you had me read and tell?

Perhaps it was the people you touched, the friends you made;

how you loved to dance and play. I think that it was all of these, but more.

It was how you loved us that remains with me today.

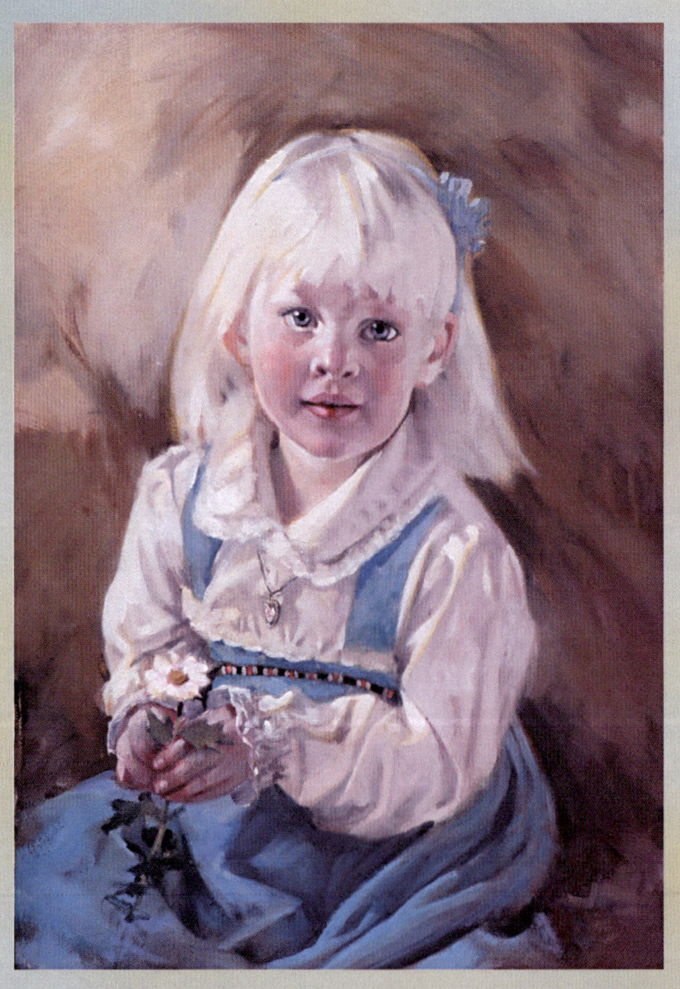

Is she really gone? No – it seemed so once.

In an effort of two worlds to unite,
my spirit like a dove takes flight.
Only when worldly illusions cease
do I soar into heaven's peace.

I can hear rippling waters telling me she is near.

I can smell pastures. The surrounding tones
change to the color she held dear.

I can see trees dancing with her as her life grows.

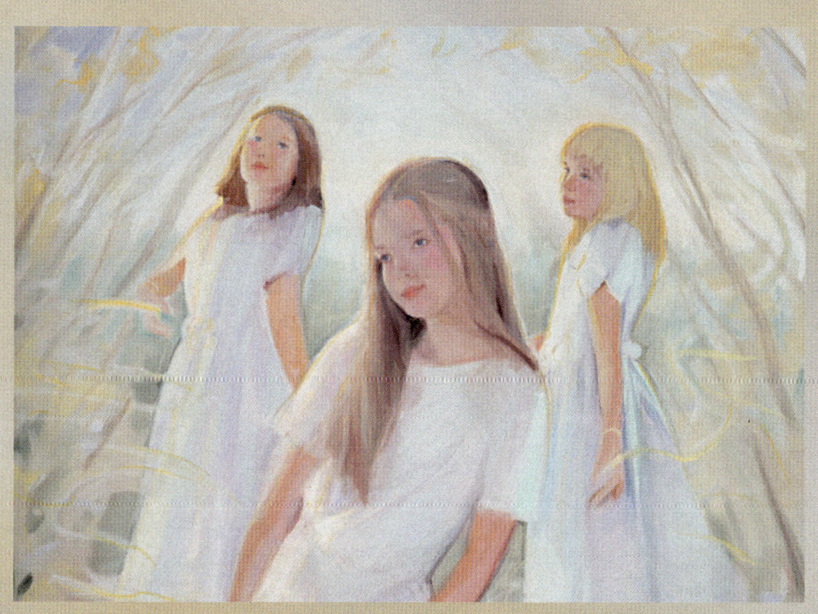

I can see mountains rising,
proclaiming the One who made her glow.

There was a time when she was gone;

now we have a son.

Yet her love for him already has begun.

When I think of you, I feel your warmth;
like the sun it never cools.
When I think of you I feel your spirit;
like the sun it never fades.

I can hear her laughter,
and the music to which she sings.
It is I who hear the stories that now,
to me, she brings.

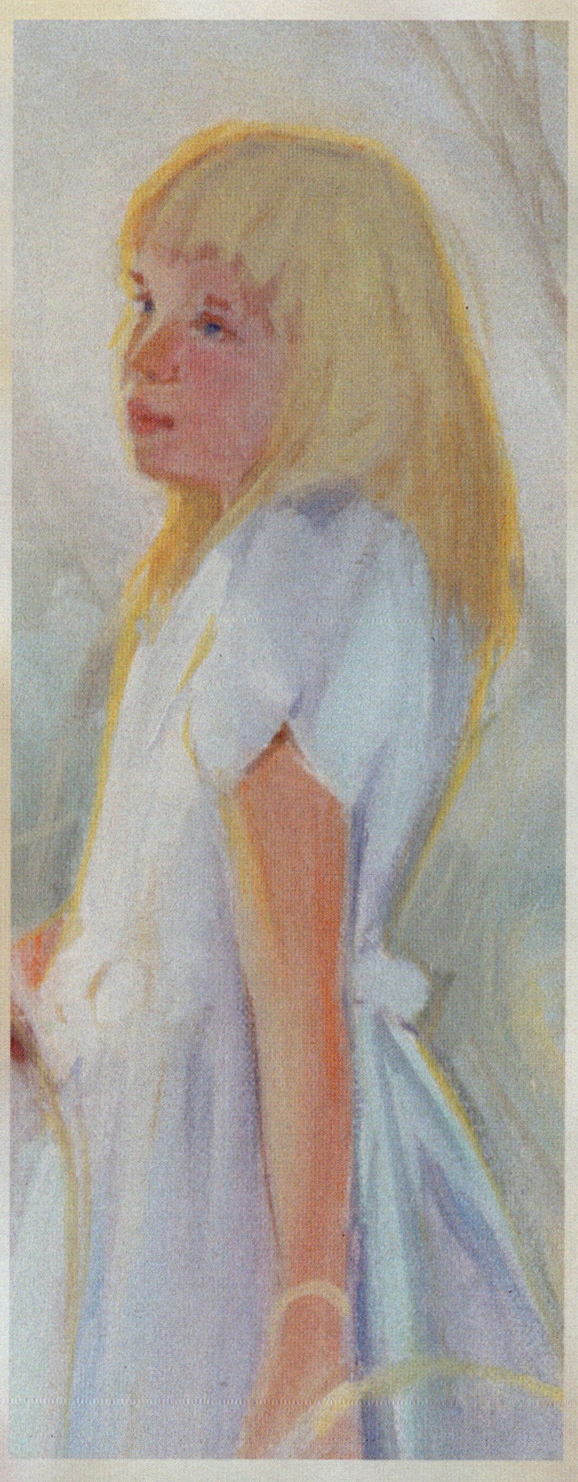

My son Ryan was four years old when I
painted this picture of him. I remember
wondering what dreams he had and would
have; what choices he would make and
what he would become.

Battles at play are fantasy. There is
always a warrior figure, a hero, someone
to emulate and look up to.

Life is compiled from many trials and
challenges. The outcome of the trials and
challenges, and what we choose as a
result of them, is who we become.

The Lord is continually presenting some
facet of Himself to us. The simplicity of the
"hero" and good against evil is perhaps
the oldest facet.

This is the theme behind this painting.

Shiloh

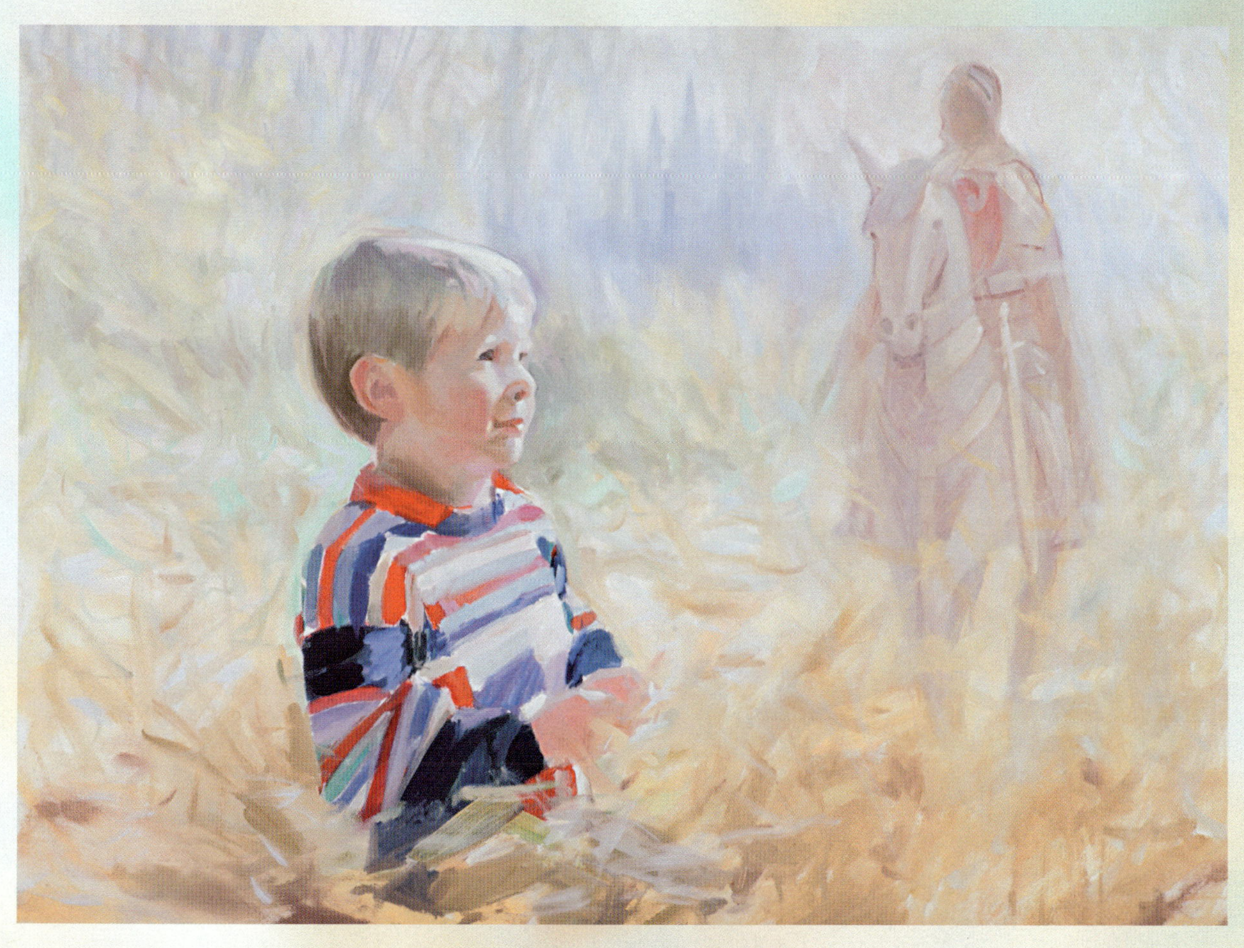

Childhood games of battle
are won, not lost.
No quest is too great,
no risk in combat too big a cost.
Defense is sure, as the eagle
is your standard.
How can one so young,
so innocent, fight single-handed?

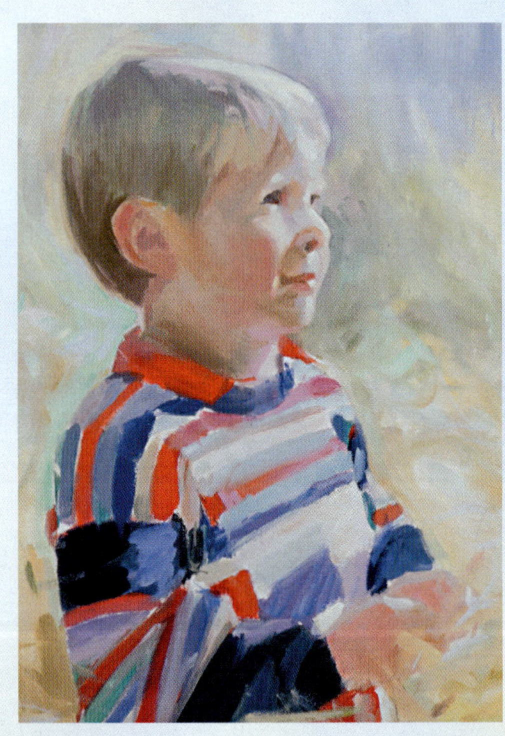

You know the fight is good against evil,
and those who confront you flee from peril.
You share in triumph your noble deed
as you return uninjured
upon your great white steed.

The world is a dream and life is a game;
but beware, child – there is a foe much greater.
He is called "Growing Up" and "Disillusionment."
And once you awaken from the dream, life is not the same.

Now we fear to fight the foe.
Now we fear to fight the battle.
Where once the smell of victory was clear,
we have built fences, but they are small defenses.

Only when injured and hungry do
we seek to regain the power of the
shield and standard.

When life and legend tune together,
with distant victory trumpets,
does the warrior return to fight in glory?
But I never knew his name was "Shiloh,"
and the game and the dream
more than a childhood story.

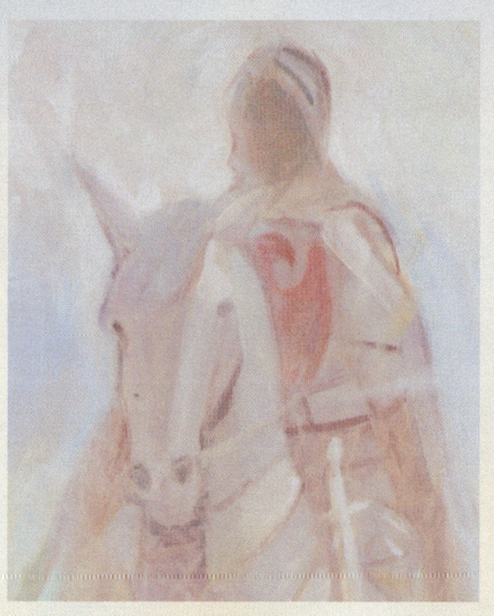

It is a dream of many of us to stay young, to
have no care in the world, or to have the hour
hand stand still. If only we could take that elixir
of eternal youth, or retreat to Shangri-La!

Are we foolish to look for a hidden paradise
or to hope for things we cannot change?
Perhaps. But it is where we go, what we are
looking for, and what we become that deter-
mines whether we will be successful.

When I was five, my mother told me that anything was possible. "Anything?" I asked.

"Anything," she replied.

As hard as I thought about it, I still couldn't fly.
Yet the fact that I failed to make the idea of
anything being possible work for me did not
stop me from believing it was true.

Eternal youth is a state of mind and the
Shangri-La, the hidden paradise, takes a lifetime to approach if it is where we want to go.

Moment in Time

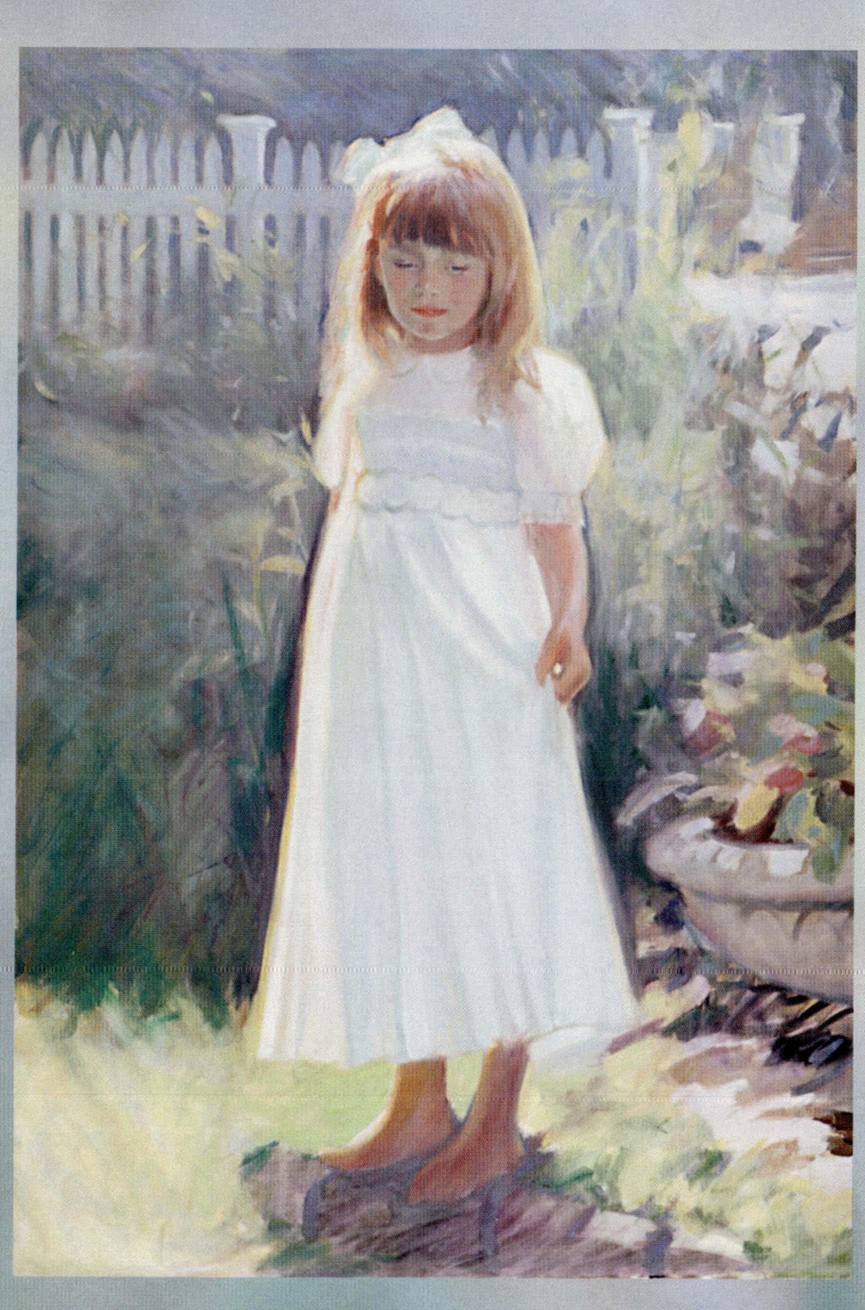

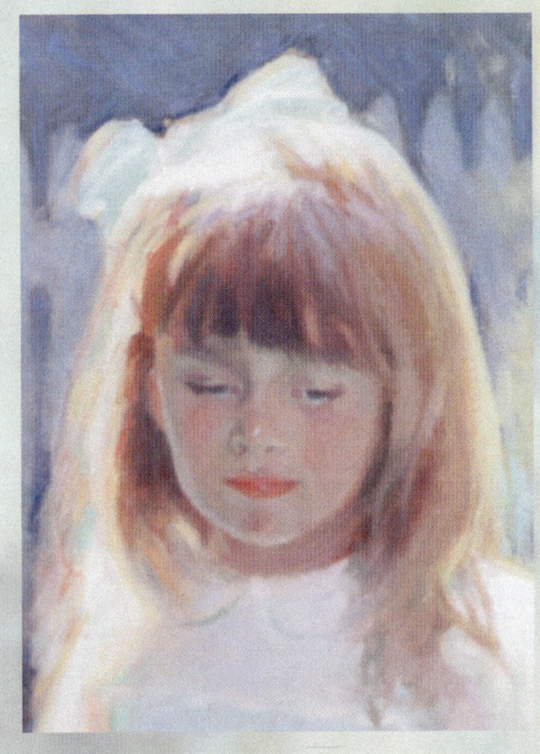

Who are you, and which way will you go?
The dreams you have will point the way.

The sun shines high; there is no shadow.
There is time to stand and stare;
cares, if at all, are only mellow.

Your dress of white reveals a true reflection
of all surrounding colors.

Captured in time and with time to spare,
you take a pensive pose;
but there is no hurry. The sun is still high
and there still is no shadow.

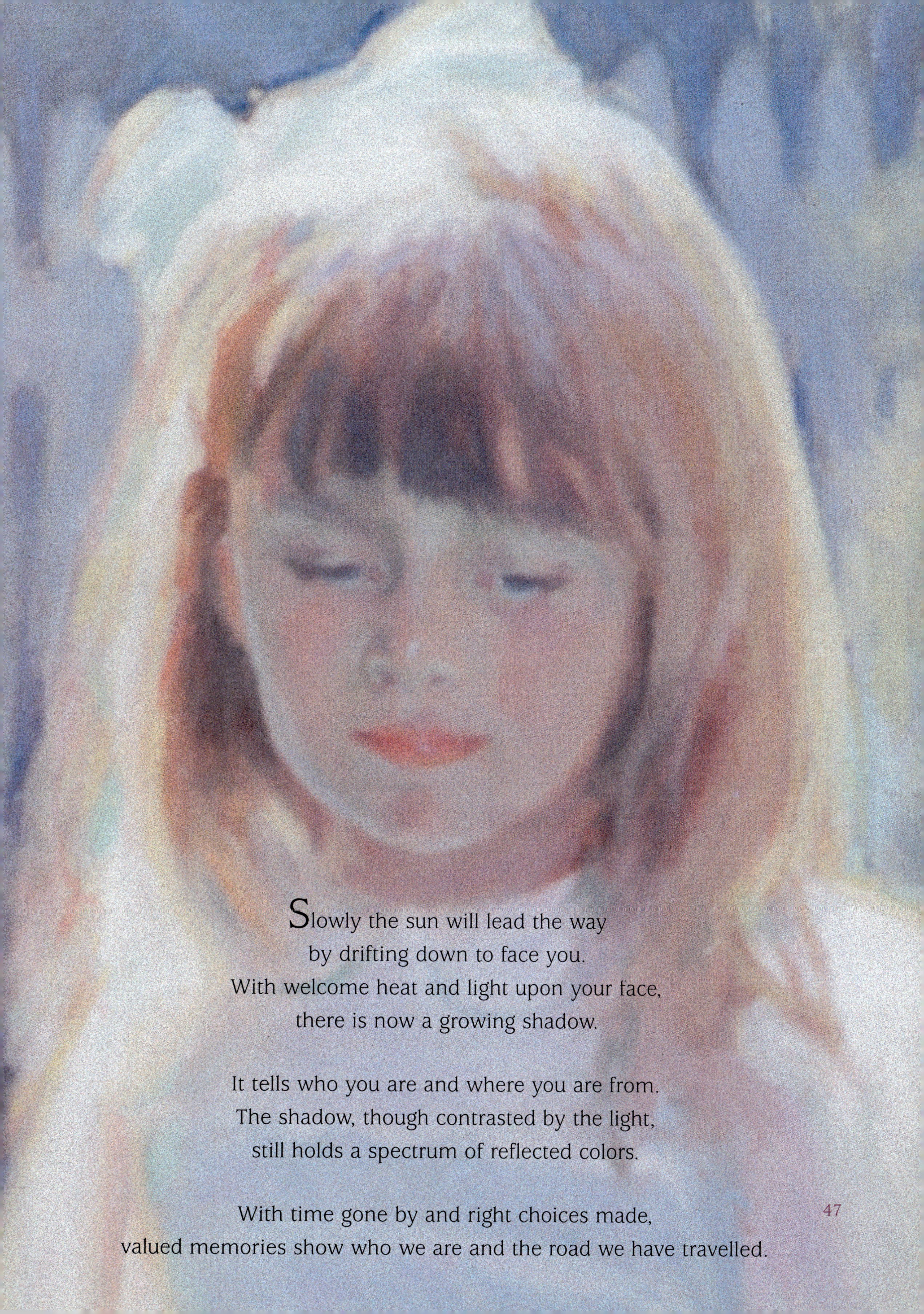

Slowly the sun will lead the way
by drifting down to face you.
With welcome heat and light upon your face,
there is now a growing shadow.

It tells who you are and where you are from.
The shadow, though contrasted by the light,
still holds a spectrum of reflected colors.

With time gone by and right choices made,
valued memories show who we are and the road we have travelled.

Have you ever wondered, as I have for
some time, what it must have been like for
John to have the Holy City there before him,
descending from God out of heaven (Rev. 21)?
There was no mistake; this was to be a place
where there would be no more pain, suffering
or darkness because it had the glory of God.
I wonder what this looked like for John. I do
know that each person, given the opportunity,
would have seen this city a little differently.
After all, the city is said to have twelve
gates or entrances.

The Holy City

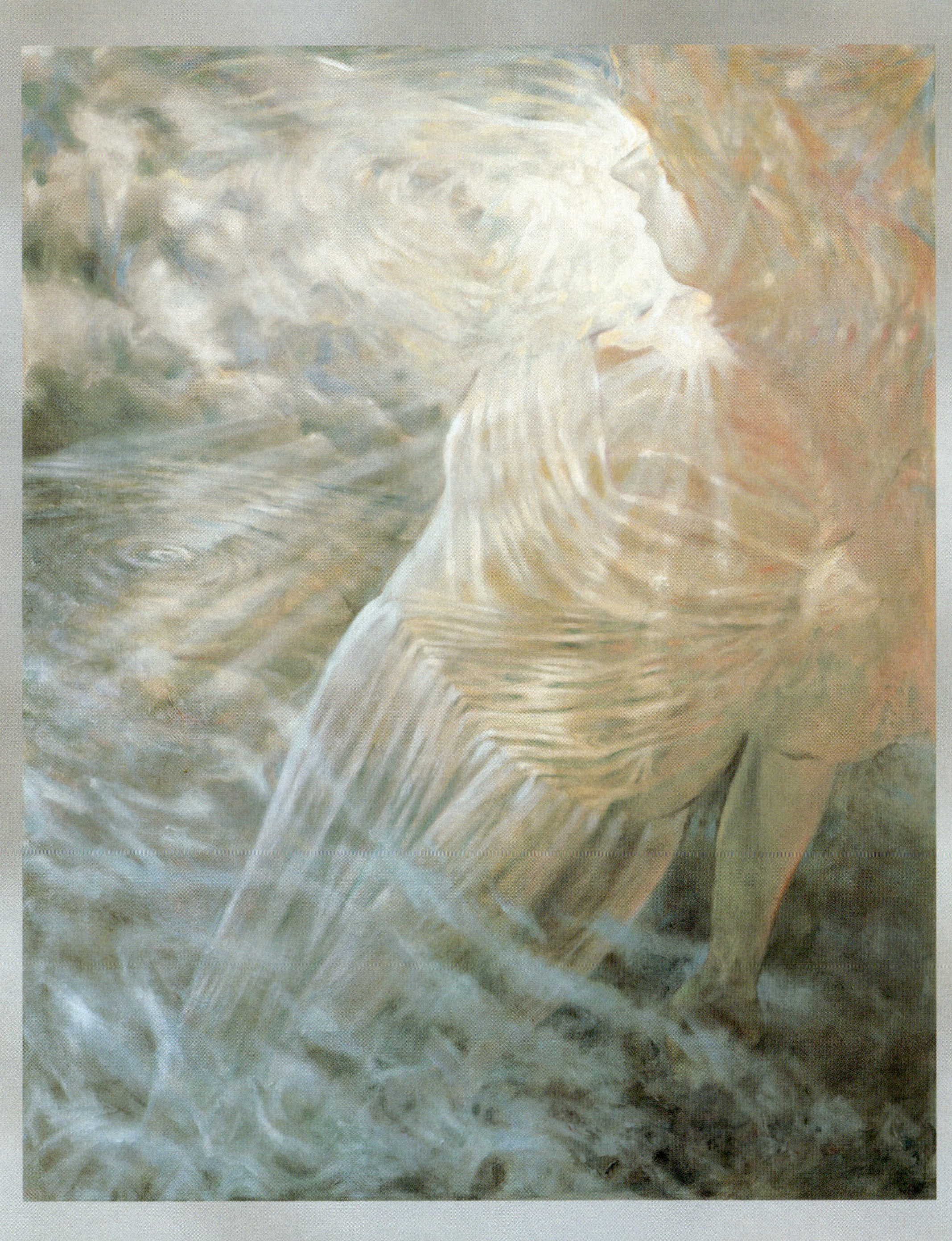

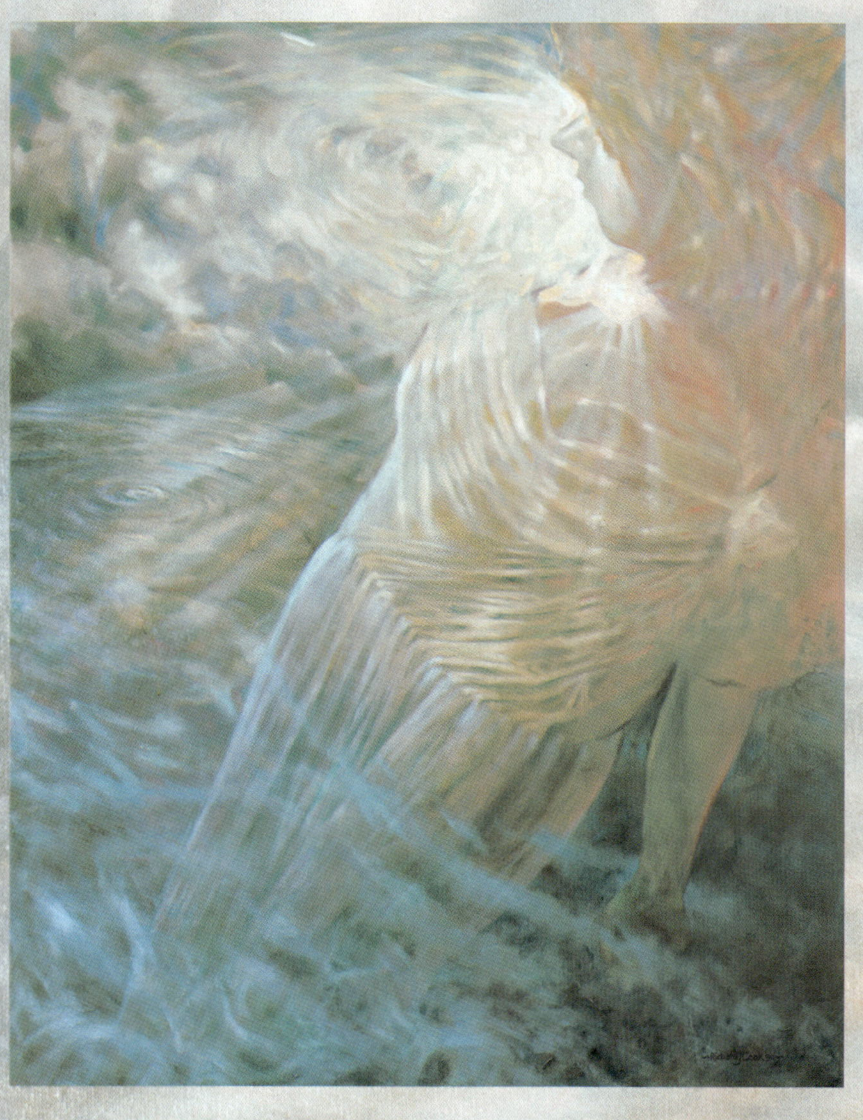

Through the Holy and transparent human form
mountains are visible, and many rivers that
converge to cascade as waterfalls.
The waterfalls disappear into darkness,
just like our lives when we doubt
and turn away from our Creator.
But these waters will eventually consume doubt
and announce a new age on earth. The waters
descend as a wall, brightly colored as jasper.

The light has two forms: light within and light without.
The light without shows man's reception of the Lord – never constant
but revolving and fluctuating, as clouds moving across the sky,
intercepting the light's passage. The light within is direct and reflects
the unchanging, consistent nature of infinite wisdom. The gold in the
city reflects the warmth of infinite love.

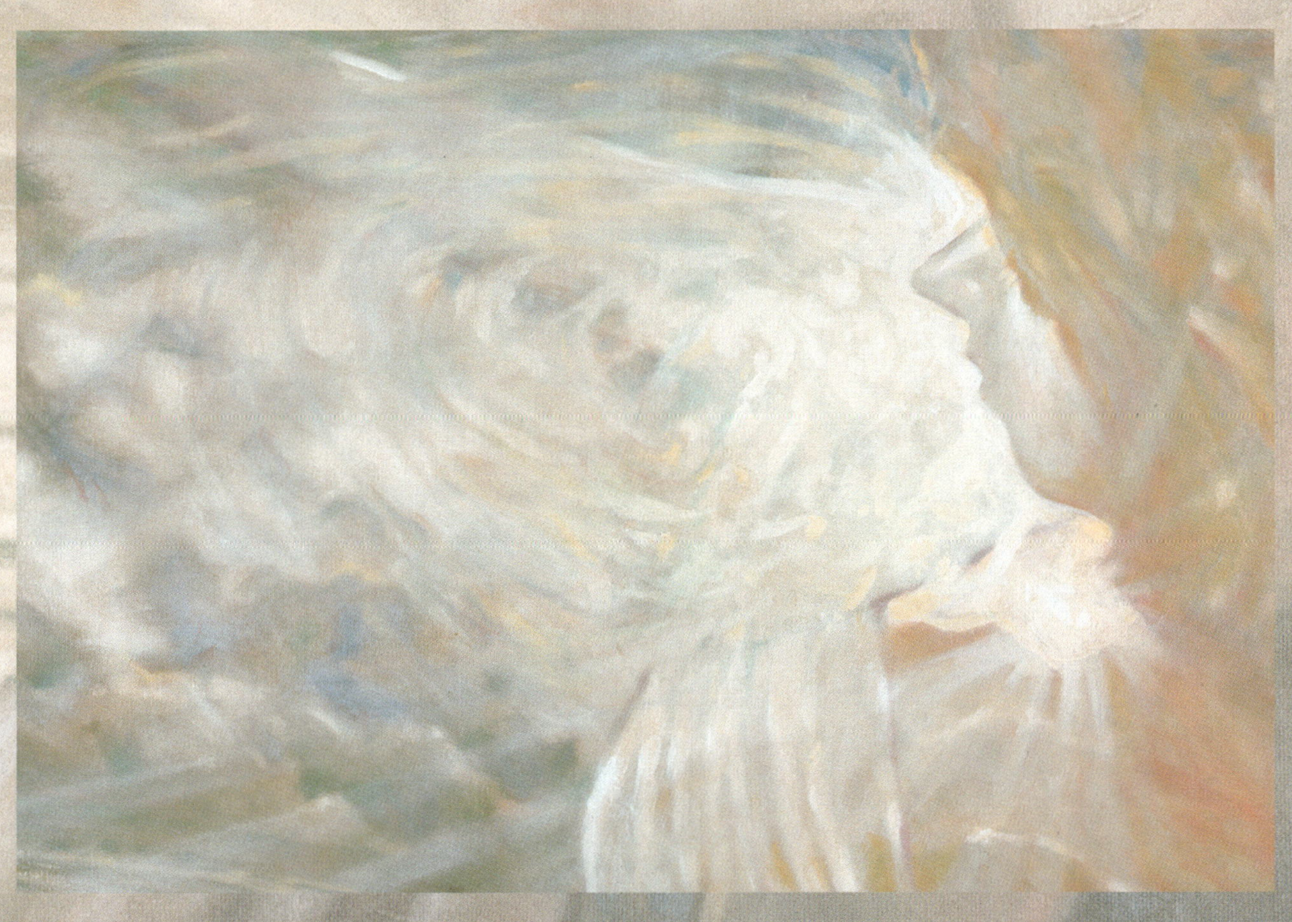

The eye of the storm is the passage by which the Lord can break
through our rage of confusion,
enabling us to look up, allowing the
realities of the world to give way to
the light of spiritual reality. It is
also the vortex through which all
travel upon death, like a tunnel or
interior wall becoming brightly colored as it ascends to the light – like
a canal to rebirth.

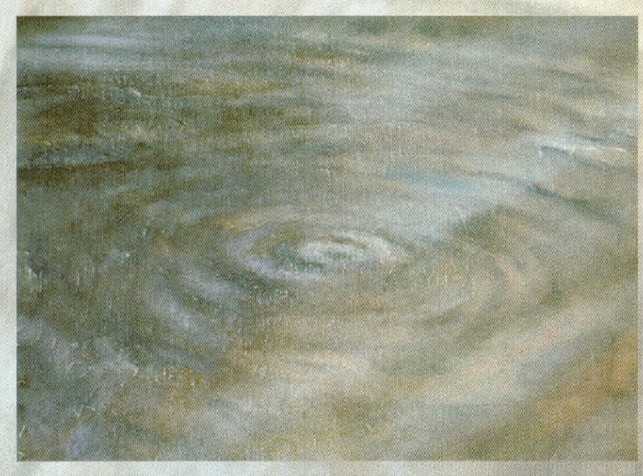

The dual process is apparent. The
Lord is constant, descending upon
our lives with purpose, to have us
ascend to His Holy City.

Then I, John, saw the holy city, New Jerusalem, coming down

from God out of heaven, prepared as a bride

adorned for her husband. Revelation 21:2

Then he measured its wall...according to the measure of a man,

that is, of an angel. And the construction of its wall was of jasper;

and the city was pure gold, like clear glass. Revelation 21:17,18

And he showed me a pure river of water of life,

clear as crystal, proceeding out

of the throne of God... Revelation 22:1

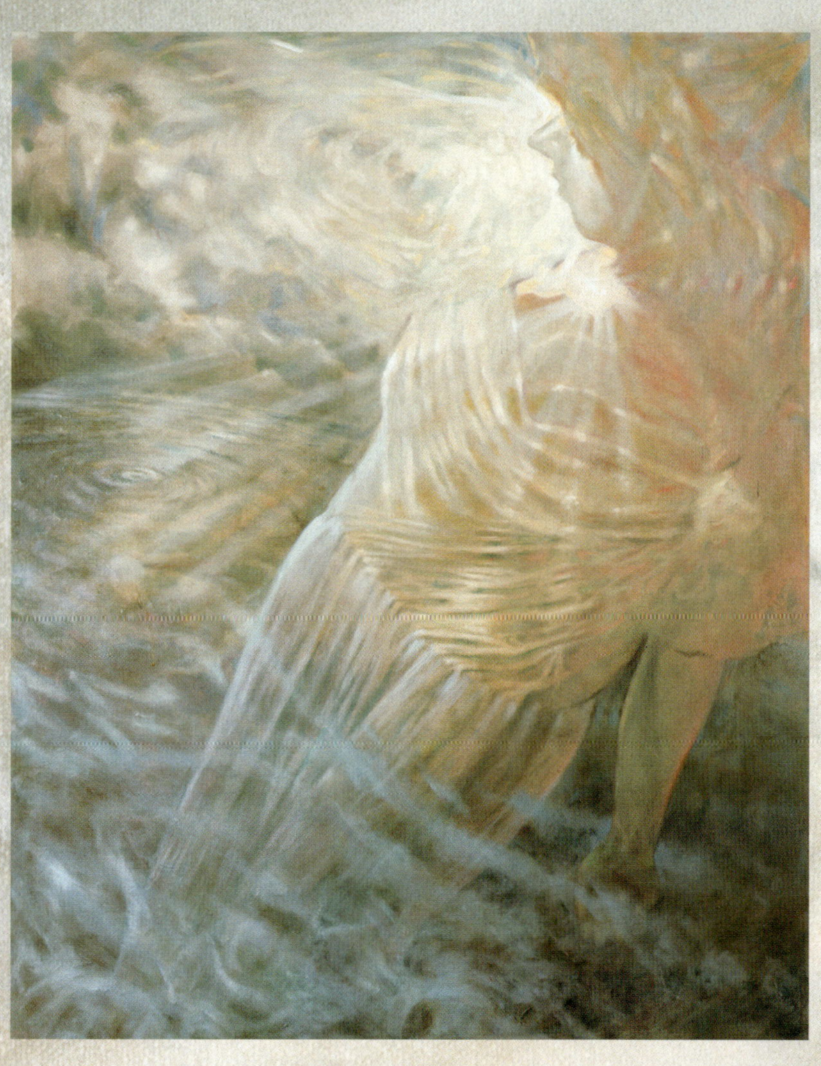

"Hummingbird" was inspired by a husband and wife who were also good friends of mine. I was always struck by their constant efforts to be useful, and to look for the good in those around them. I looked at their inspiring optimism, their hunger to be useful and their love for the Lord.

When trying to picture these qualities I saw in my mind a hummingbird. There is an ancient Aztec story of a dance where the men lift the women above their heads, and they are said to turn into hummingbirds and fly. Why this metamorphosis?

I chose these Aztec images to express the spiritual union of husband and wife performing uses together, and the metamorphosis that occurs through these uses.

Hummingbird

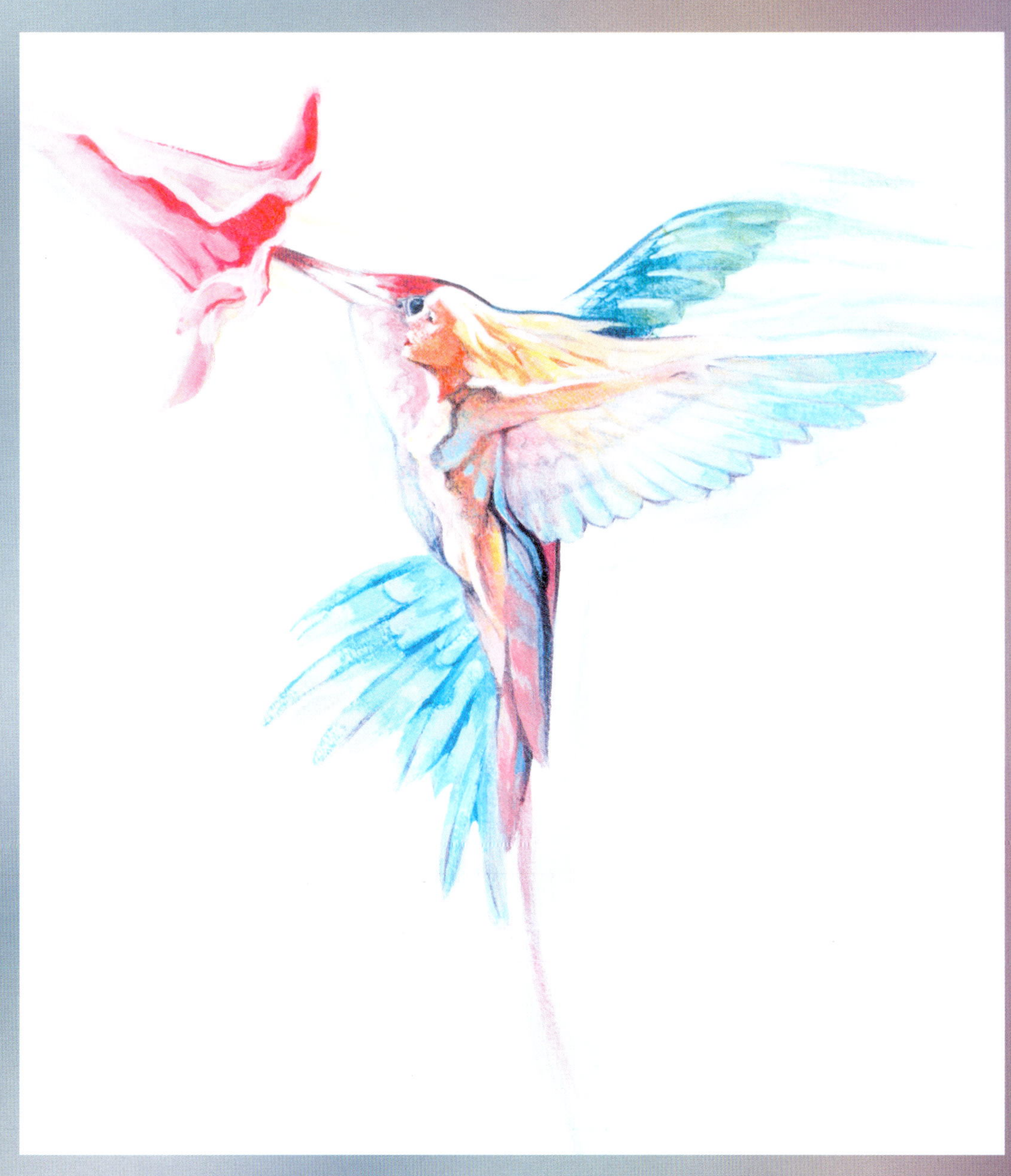

May you always feel His presence
And sense which way to turn.
You bring us joy when you are near,
Your absence begs your return.

When you drink from life's sweet waters
You hover and are gone a while.
With use and need and rapid speed
You are back to feed from the vial.

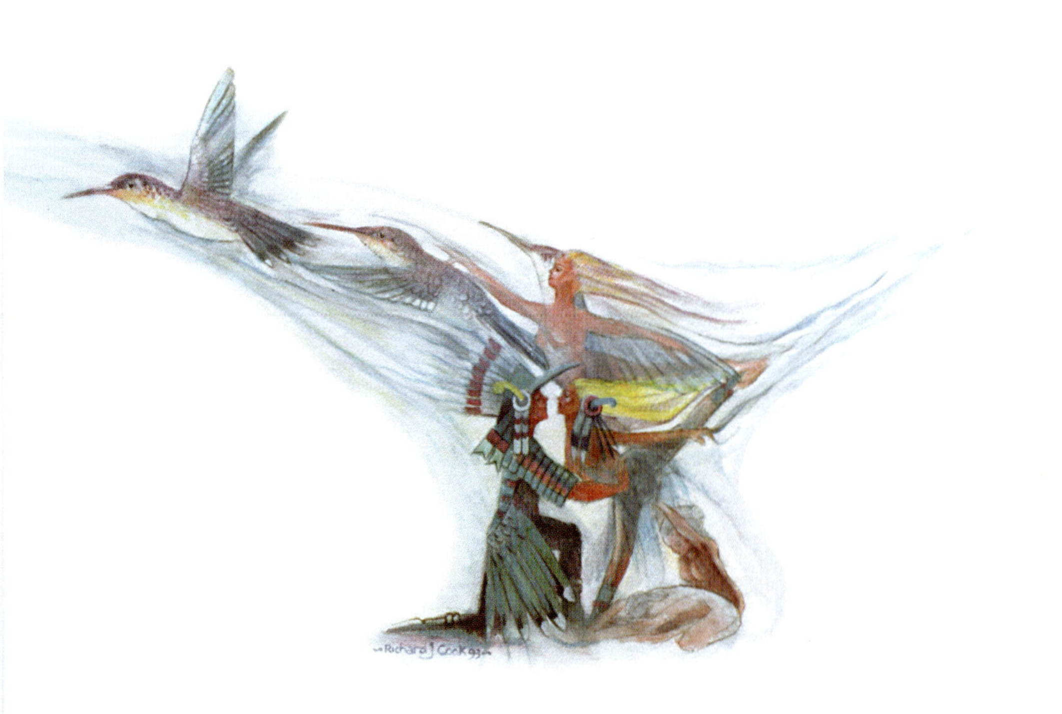

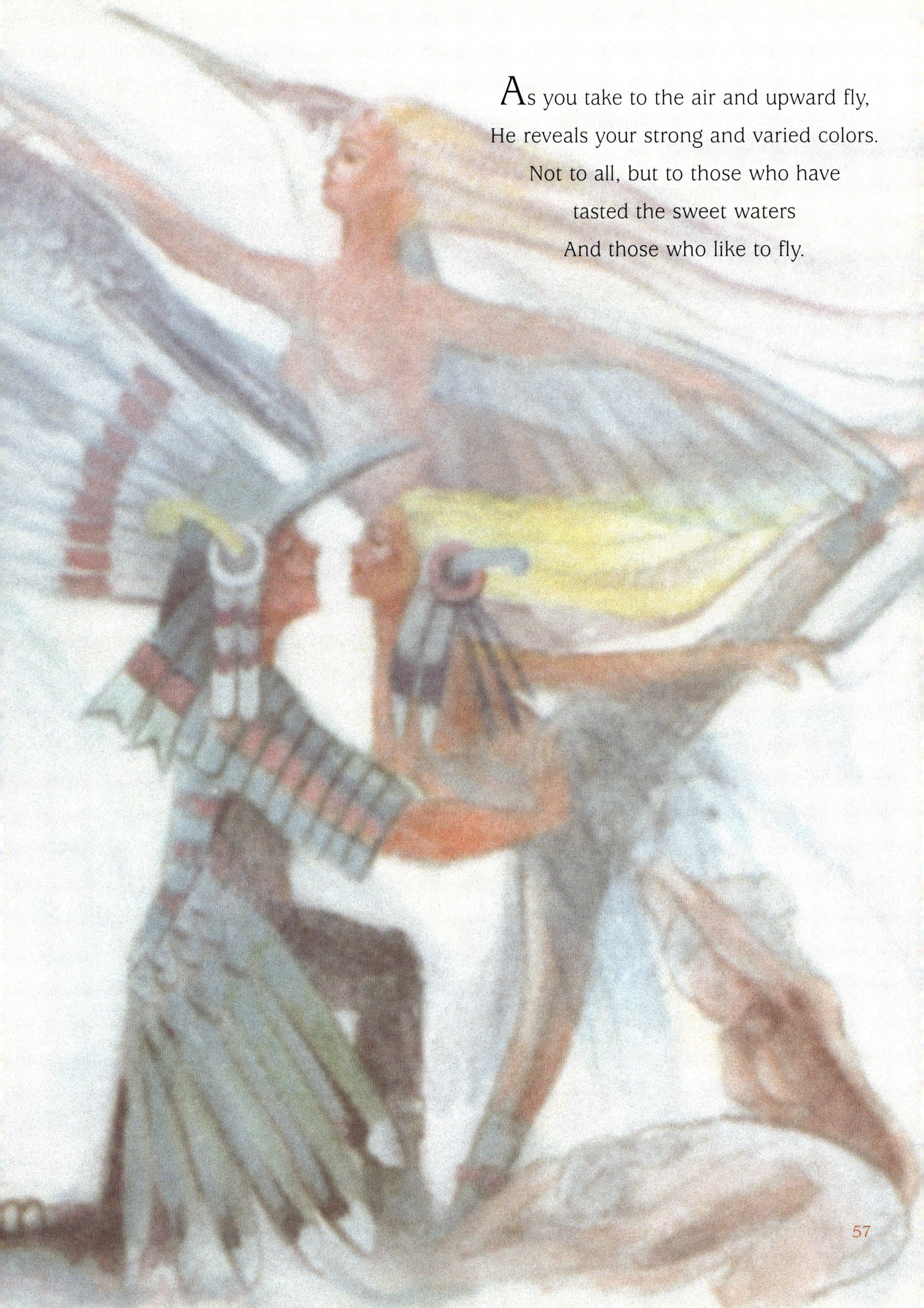

As you take to the air and upward fly,
He reveals your strong and varied colors.
Not to all, but to those who have
tasted the sweet waters
And those who like to fly.

The twenty-third Psalm has often entered
into my mind in times of spiritual conflict,
effectively comforting my soul. The woman in
this painting represents our individual lives, our
times of darkness and, with the Lord, our times
of inspiration and light. She represents our
changing confidence in the Lord. The
Shepherd, however, is always there reaching
down, constant and beckoning.

The Lord is My Shepherd

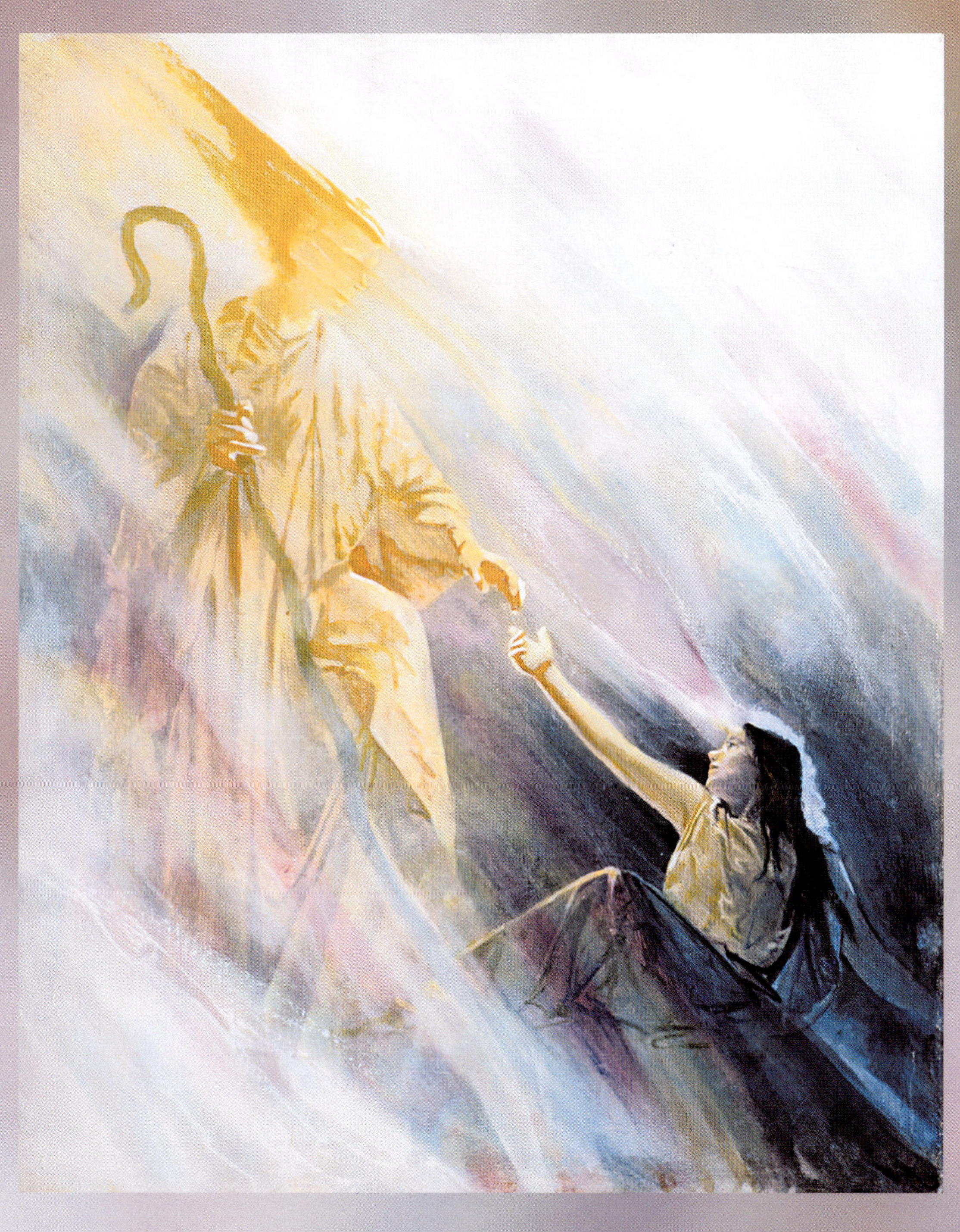

Out of my darkness I came,
My troubles great, my illusions many.
I walk in a valley of shadows
And my world is of time and space.

My darkness makes the way treacherous;
I often stumble. The path I follow is
illusive and ill-defined. Where are You?
Why are You not with me?

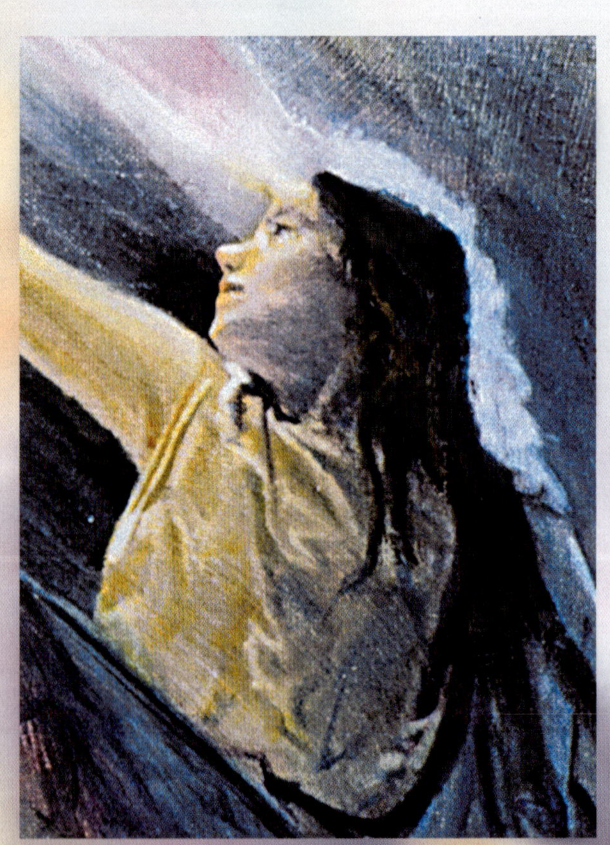

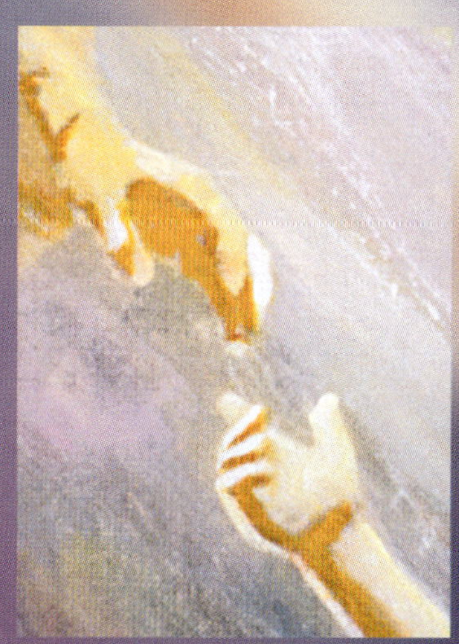

Like the seasons I revolve,
With the seasons I evolve.
Ever closer to You I reach.
The strain gives way to peace
And the touch of Your fire
Has reached my desire.

You are always there,
inclined to lift me up,
Touching the core of my heart.

Yea though I walk through
the valley of the shadow of death,
I will fear no evil, for thou art with me;
thy rod and thy staff,
they comfort me.

Psalm 23:4

"Autumn Years" takes a look at old age and some of the special qualities that can exist during this time. It also attempts to draw a parallel between the innocence found in young children and the innocence in old age. We are all born with this innocence, but it takes a lifetime to regain it.

Ultimately, the old saying is true: "You are as old as you feel," not necessarily as old as you look. There is a beauty in old age, and this is why I chose to use the image of leaves. Leaves are at their most stunning just as they are about to die.

Autumn Years

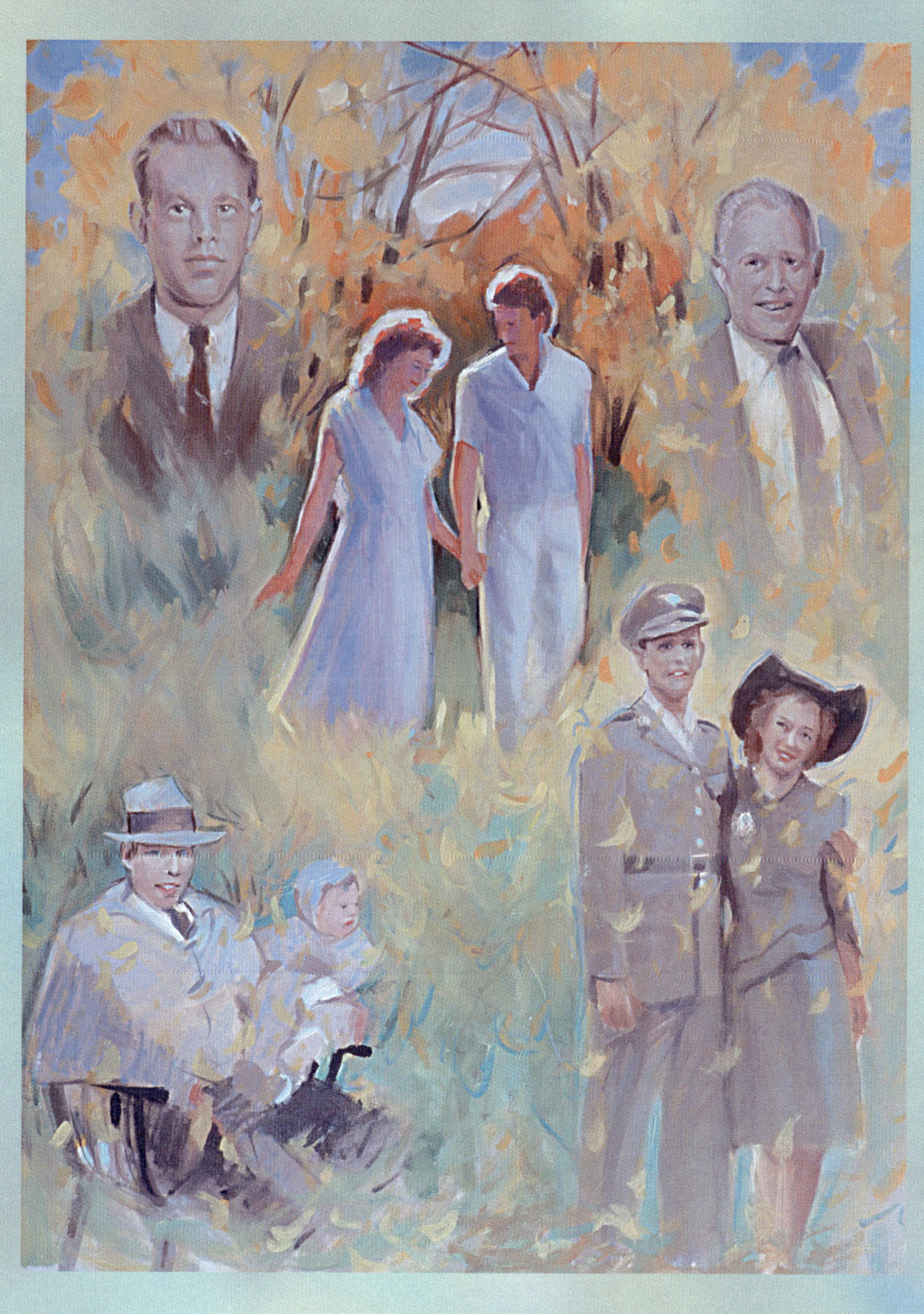

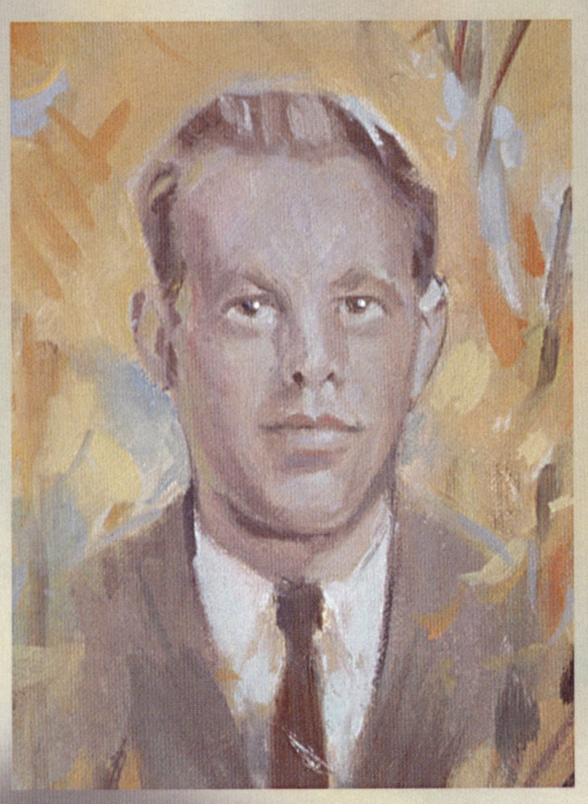

Leaves are many and varied.
Most shine in glory in their dying age.

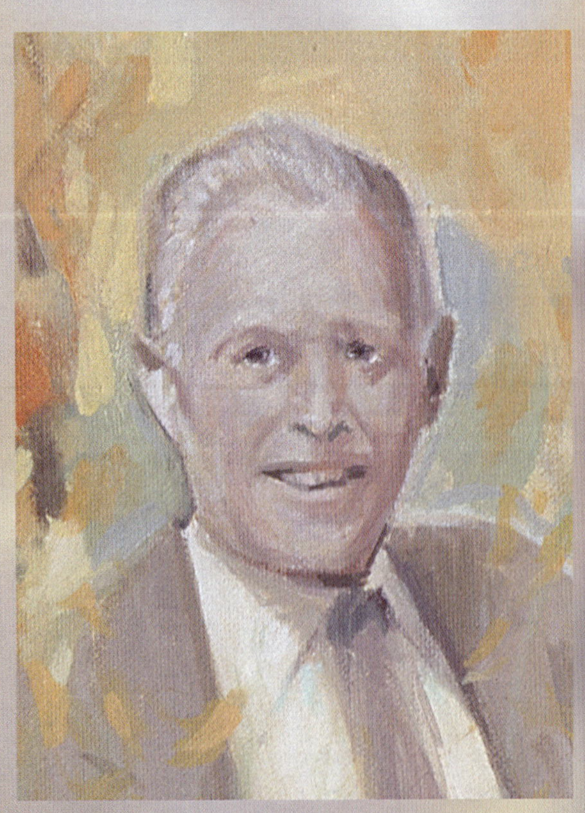

Do we look back in sorrow
as the leaves take wing to the wind?
Or perhaps in death a course is set
that leads to the promised land.

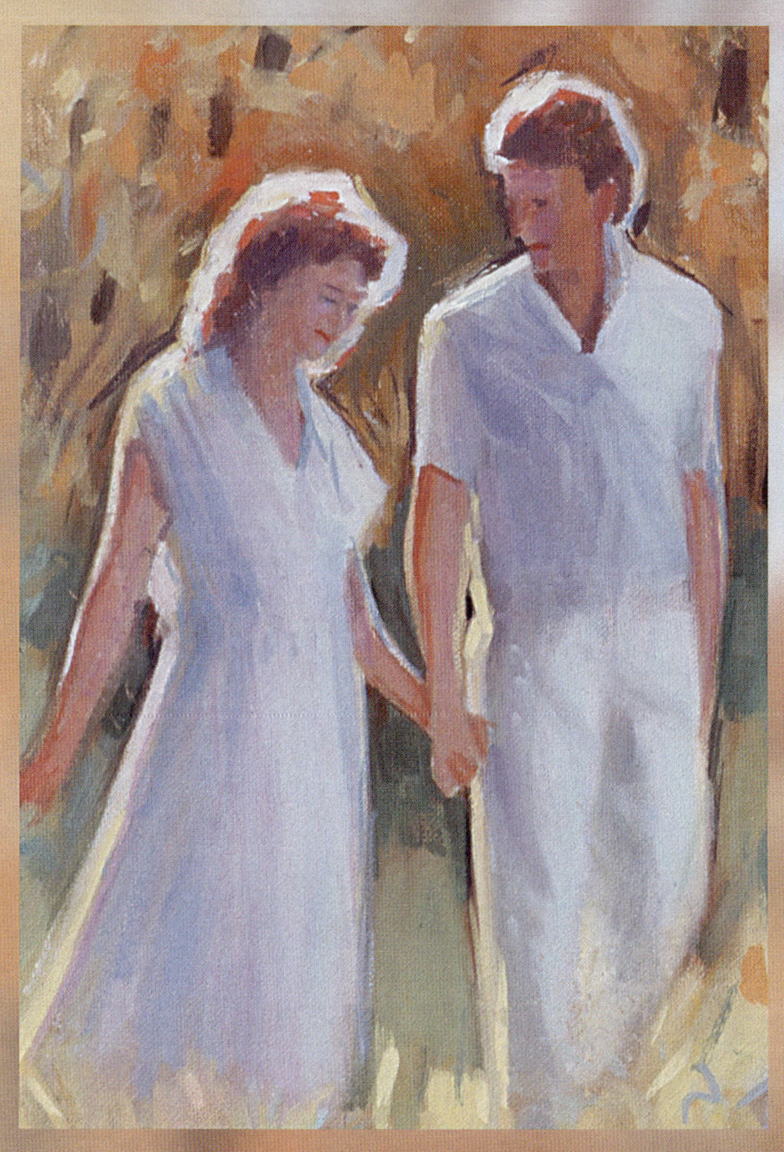

Some see only death in winter,
and some see winter as sleep.

When I have seen the autumn
colors, those treasures are
mine to keep.

And now I perceive a brave new
day, when sage and youth join in
a golden age.

Have you ever read the description in
Revelation about the woman clothed with the
sun? This passage tells of a woman who is
about to give birth. She is said to be clothed
with the sun, to have a crown of twelve stars,
and to have the moon beneath her feet.

What a powerful image! I suppose this
would need to be powerful in order for her
and the child to be protected from the great
red dragon with seven heads and ten
horns, bent on destroying.

I painted the woman clothed with the sun
in order to bring some order to these
descriptions. I excluded the dragon, as we
understand little of the perception of heaven,
but have enough evidence of the "dragon"
in the world around us.

Woman Clothed With the Sun

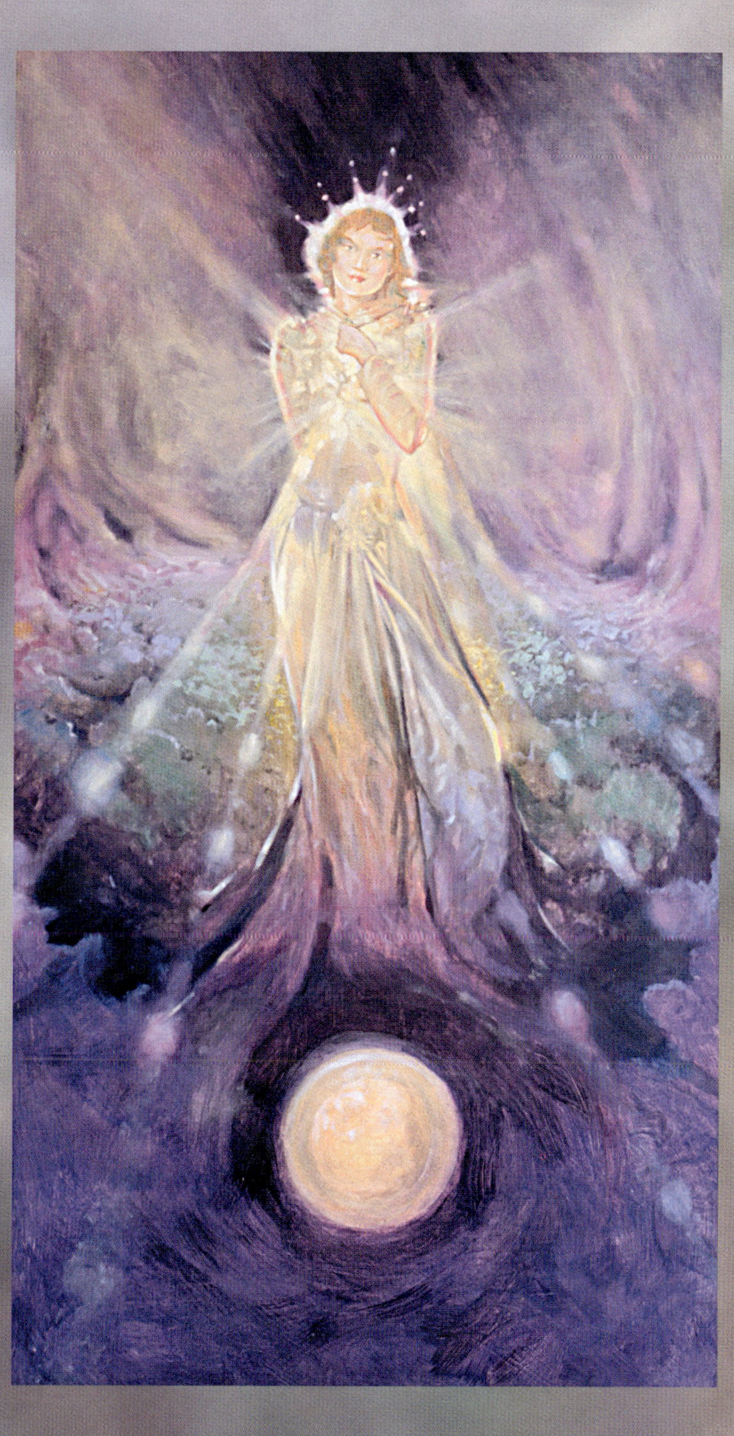

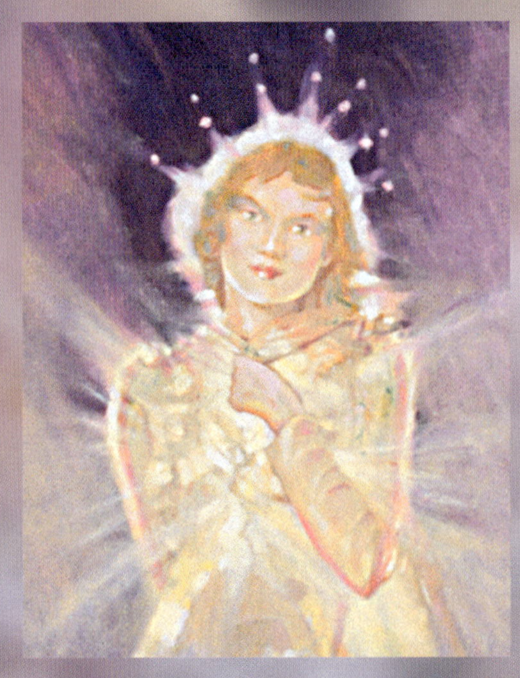

*And there appeared
a great wonder in heaven,
a woman clothed with the sun
and the moon under her feet;
and upon her head a crown of twelve stars.*

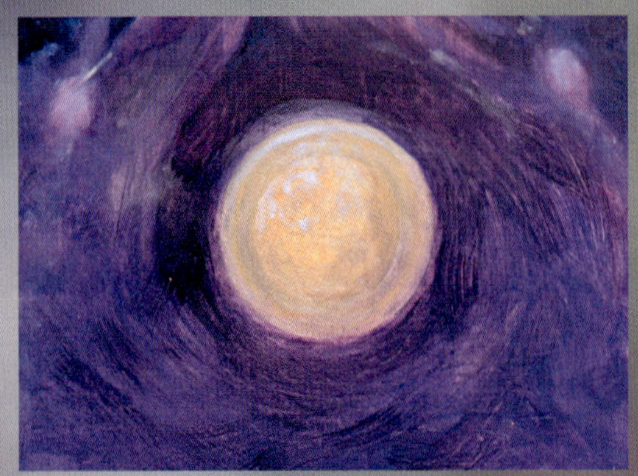

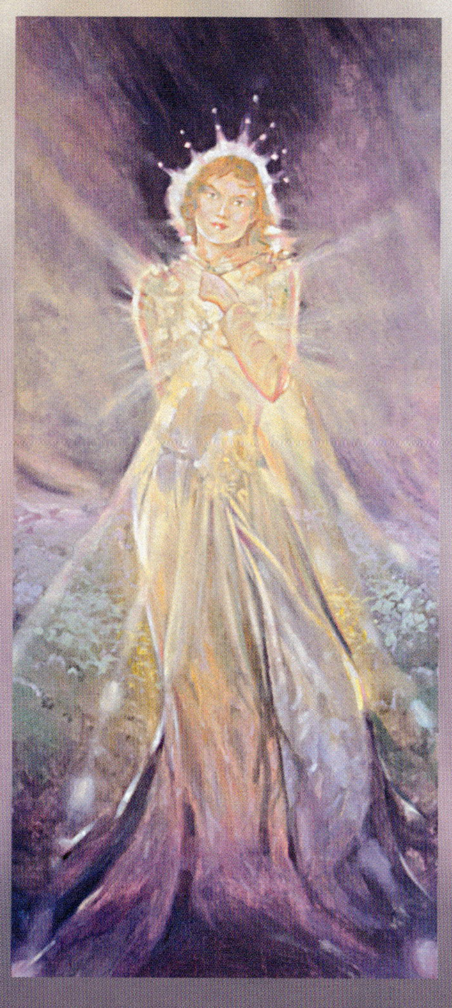

*A*nd she being with child cried,
travailing in birth, and pained to be delivered.

Revelation 12:1, 2

Thoughts leading to the making of this painting began with observations of the
people of the church that I attended. There
are two planes of growth: the outer
appearance and the inner reality.

The lower portion of the painting represents
the everyday experiences we all have with
cyclical changes of hope, fear, despair,
indifference, trust and again hope.

The upper portion of the painting is there to
represent the reality we don't necessarily see.
We are all spiritual beings and through our
experiences, with the Lord's help, we are
growing spiritually. I chose to show these same
people growing and rising as a tree.

Cedar of Lebanon

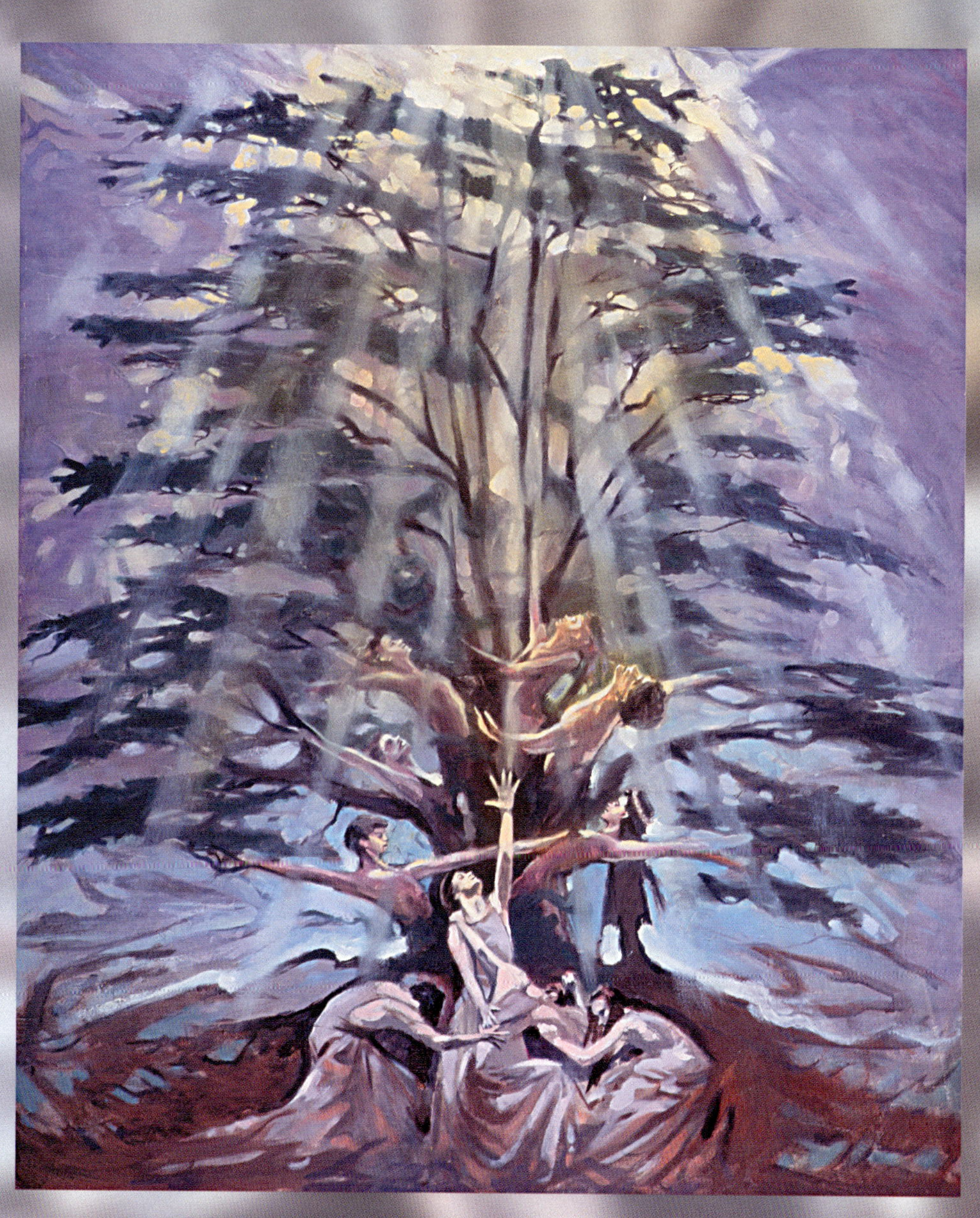

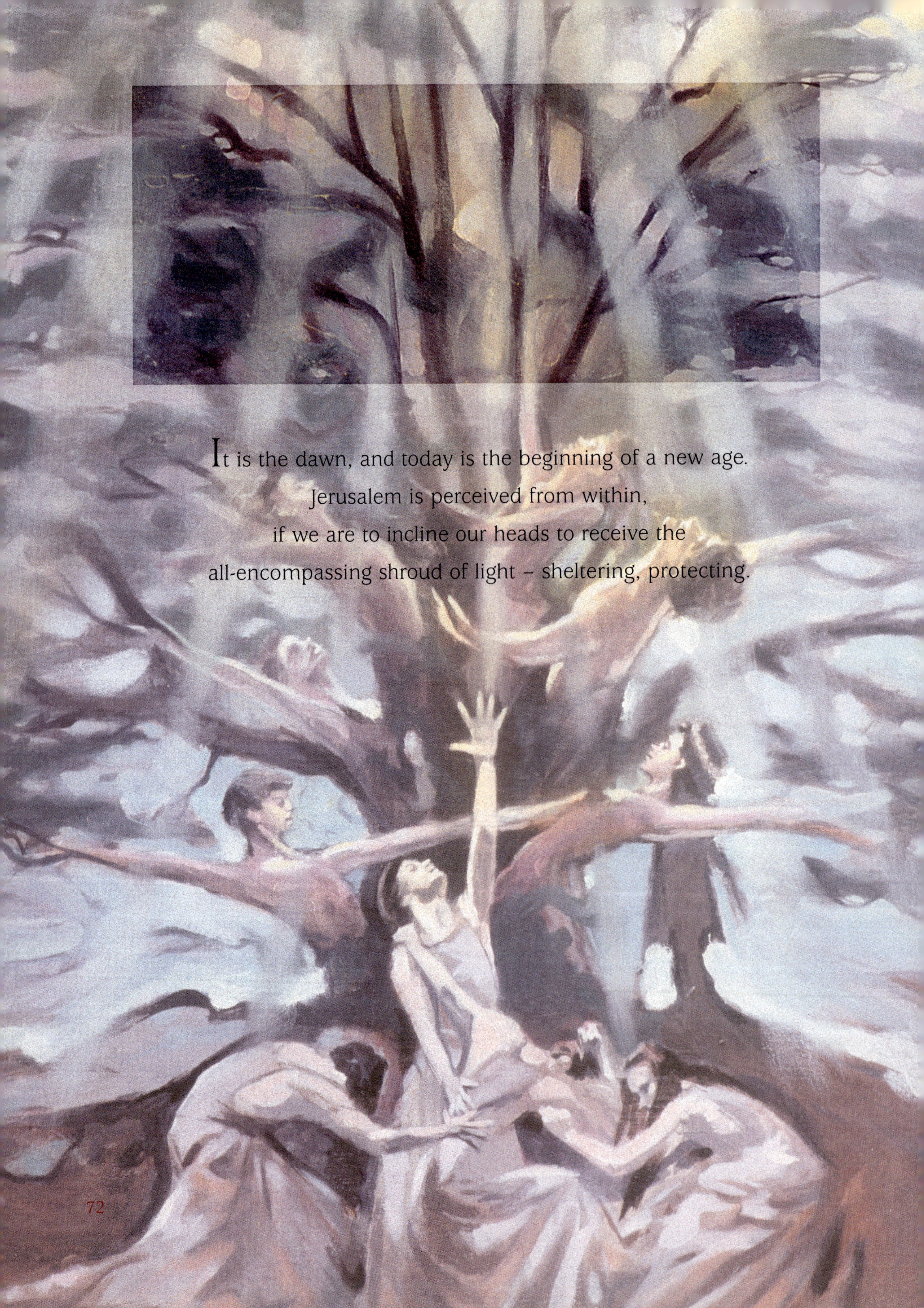

It is the dawn, and today is the beginning of a new age.
Jerusalem is perceived from within,
if we are to incline our heads to receive the
all-encompassing shroud of light – sheltering, protecting.

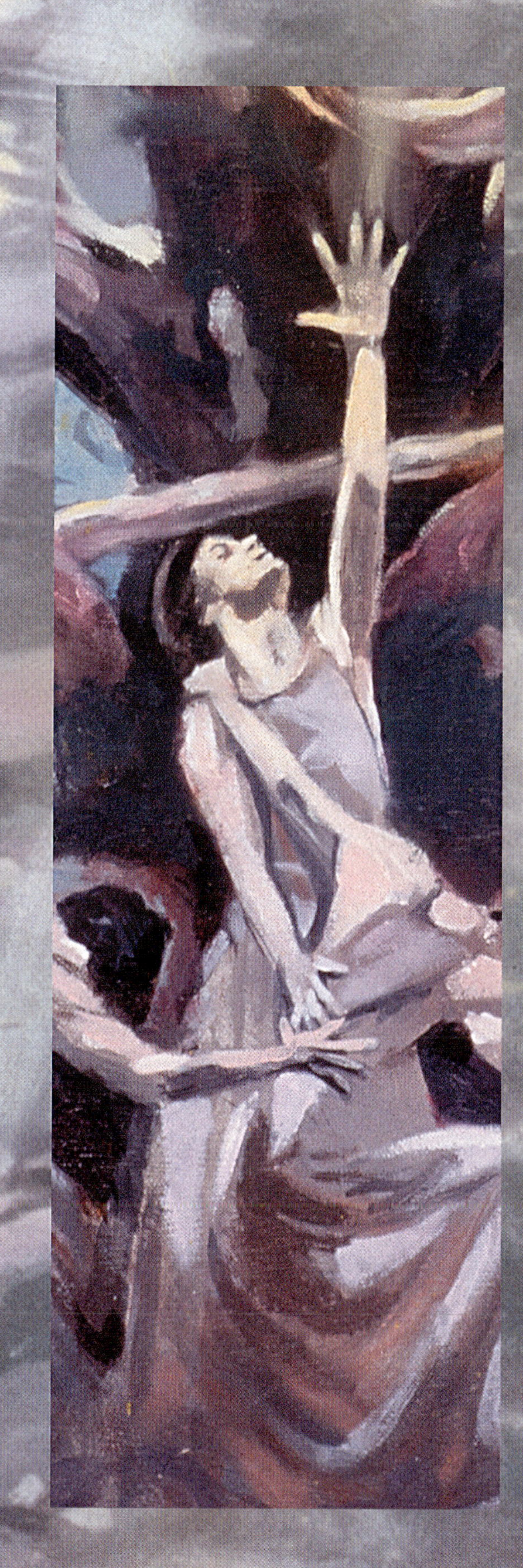

As we seek the Lord, we find strength in others, by shared friendship and compassion. We can harness this strength in times of hardship, as we also can show the way toward hope for others in their times of weakness. This fluctuation is like the ebbing tide, whose waves stroke the shore, instructed by the constant in-flowing of Divine Light.

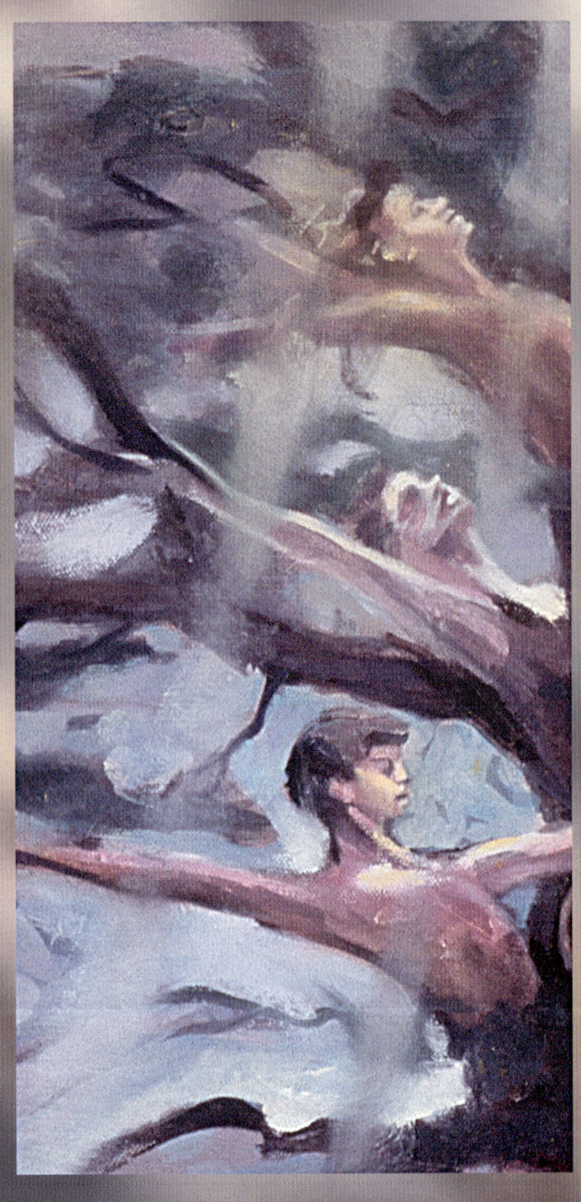

With the continuous cycles
of our life in the natural world,
we may forget our dual existence,
and with it, our ascent
into the Lord's kingdom.

The Cedar of Lebanon is the ascent of humankind,
in all our spiritual diversity, with our ability to reach up
for an ideal, and grasp the uppermost perceptions
of spiritual truth and heavenly peace.

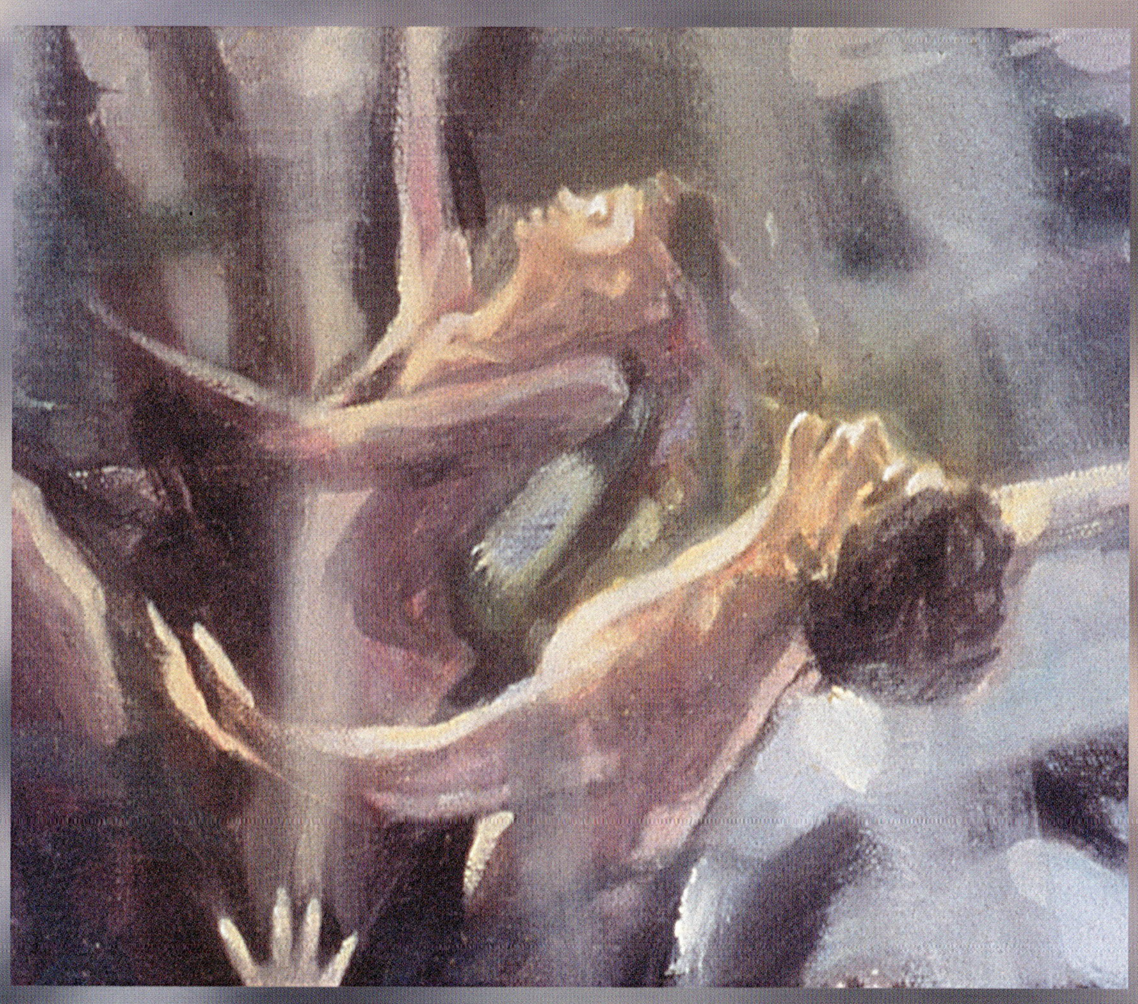

Our son Daniel was three months old, and it was a pleasure to be touched by the sphere of innocence which the Lord let us share through him. This was the inspiring spark for this painting.

Innocent Age

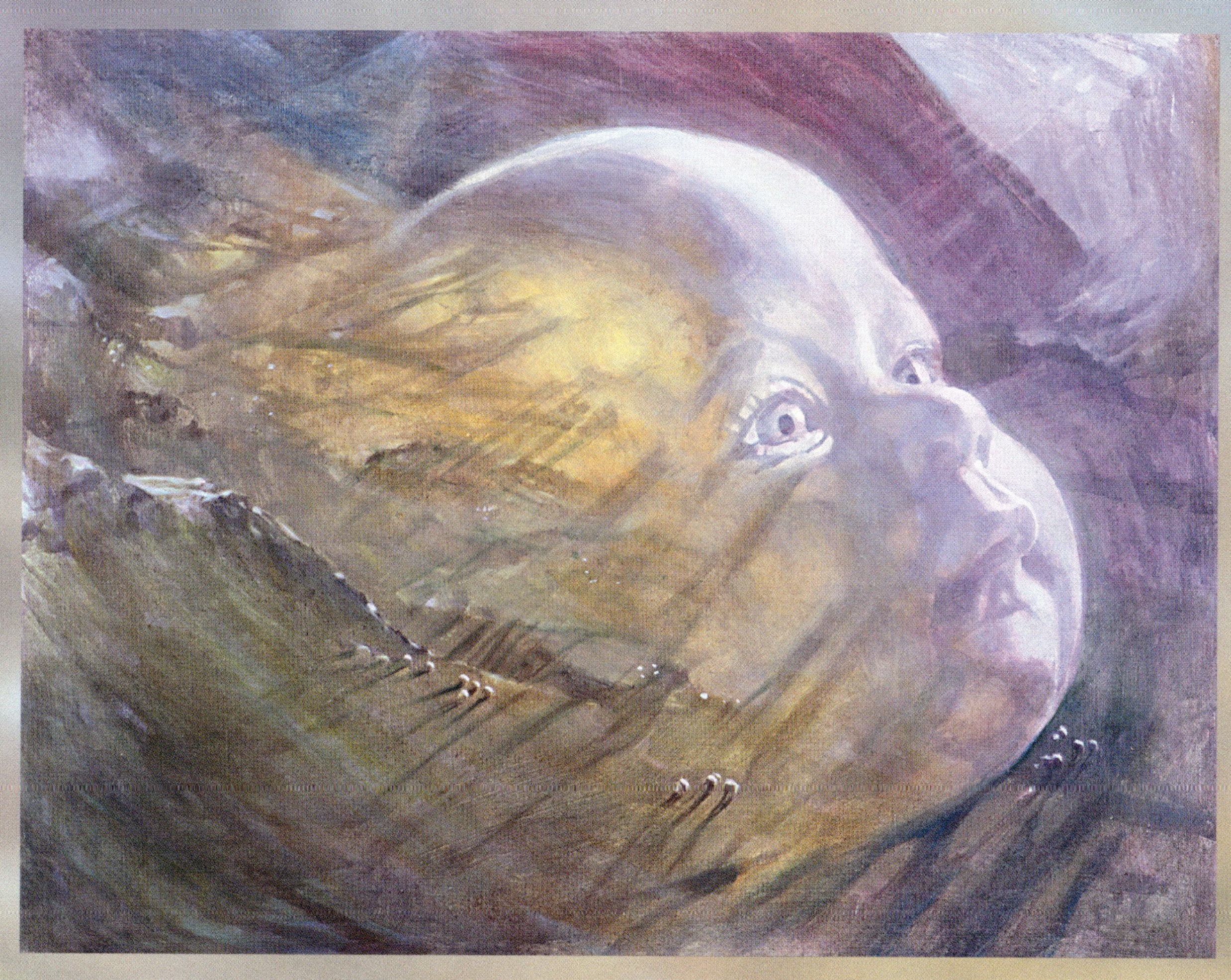

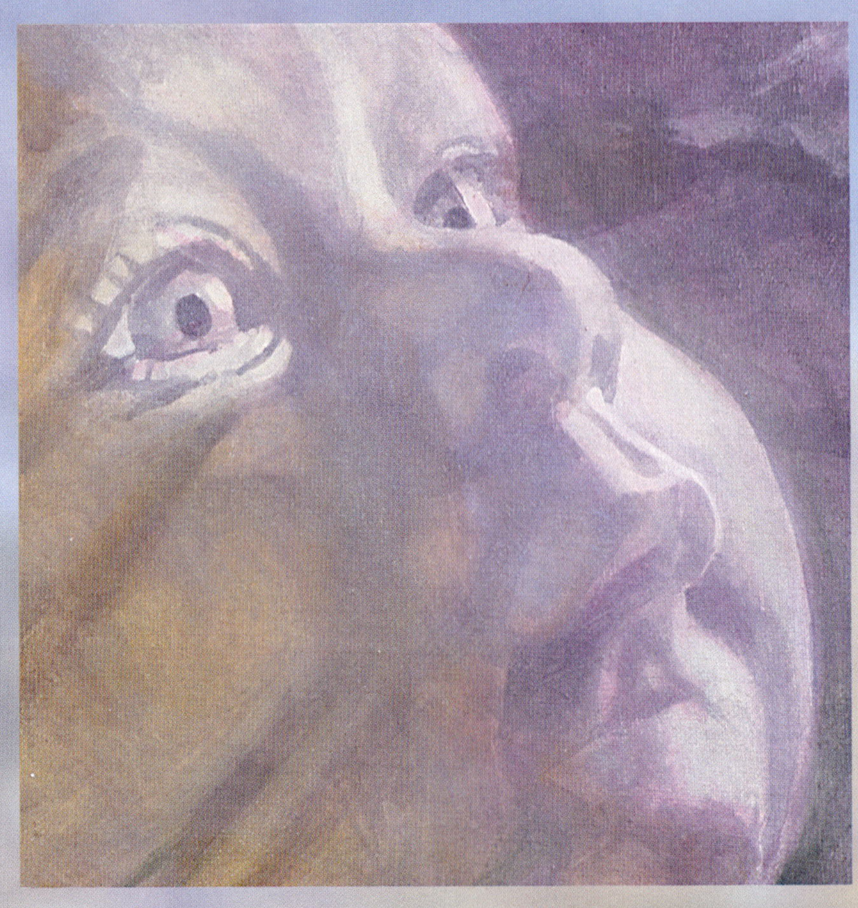

<Tender are the days of an innocent age.
You are a sign, a promise, and the answer to a prayer.

Your needs are simple, your love is sure and your
potential great. If only I could reach that state.

May the mountains protect
you from adverse winds, and
may you always ascend the hills
among the sheep and the Lamb.

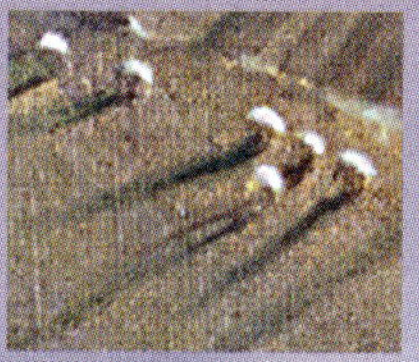

*The mountains
skipped like rams,
the little hills like lambs.*

Psalms 114:6

Judah is a lion's whelp; from the prey, my son,
thou art gone up; he stooped down,
he couched as a lion, and as an old lion;
who shall rouse him up?

The scepter shall not depart from Judah, nor a
lawgiver from between his feet, until Shiloh come;
and unto him shall be the obedience of the people.
Genesis 49:9, 10

This prophecy is most commonly attributed to the coming of the Messiah in the old Testament. The rich imagery surrounding this prophecy announces a huge event, the birth of Jesus. Can this old prophecy be talking about us now as it was then? Jesus did say to His disciples, "I will come again." Would He do this in person, or some other way? What we do know is that His coming would be the light and the way and the truth. I have always been intrigued by the words of C.S. Lewis in his "Narnia" books: "Aslan is on the move."

Crown of Glory

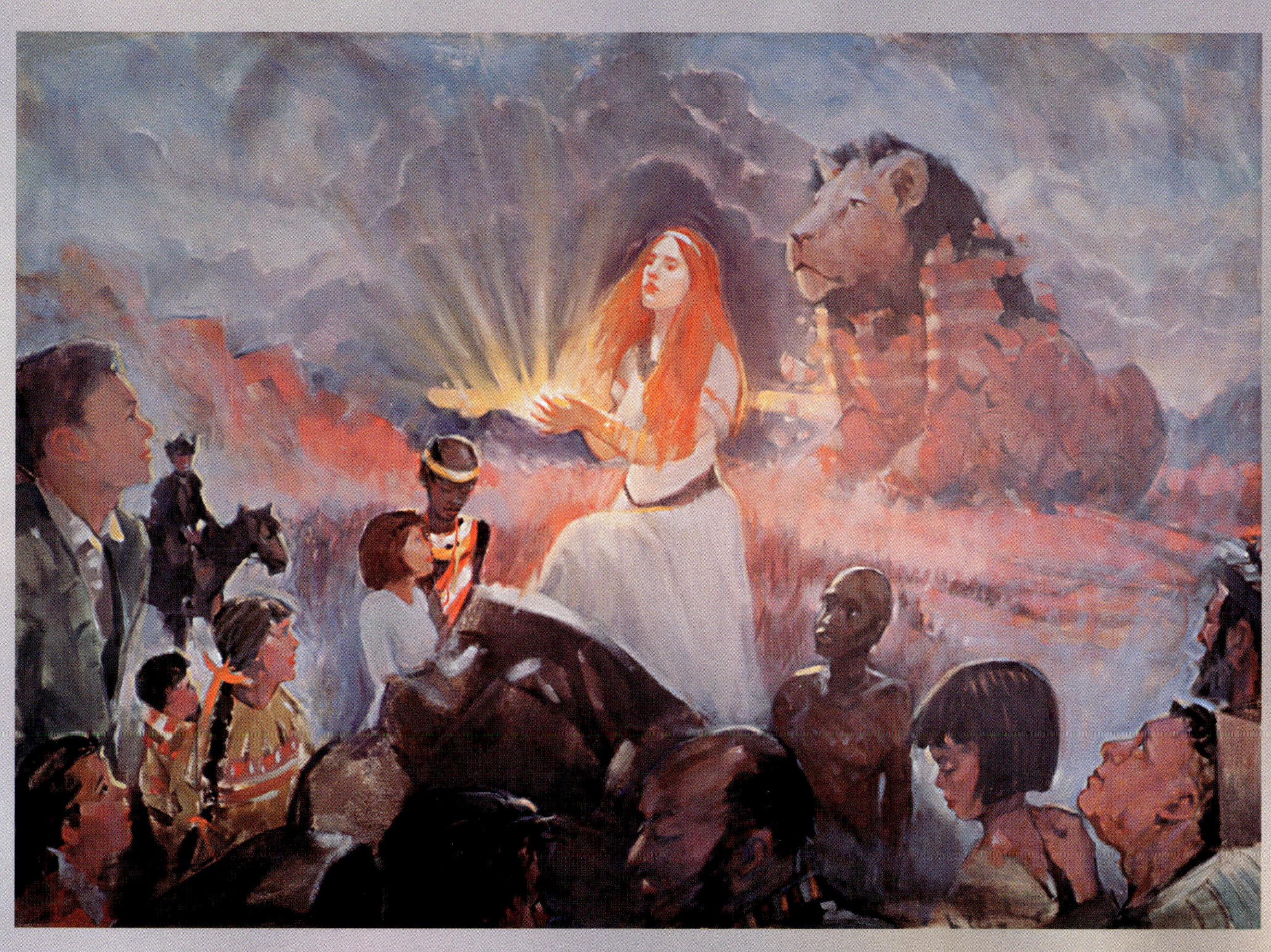

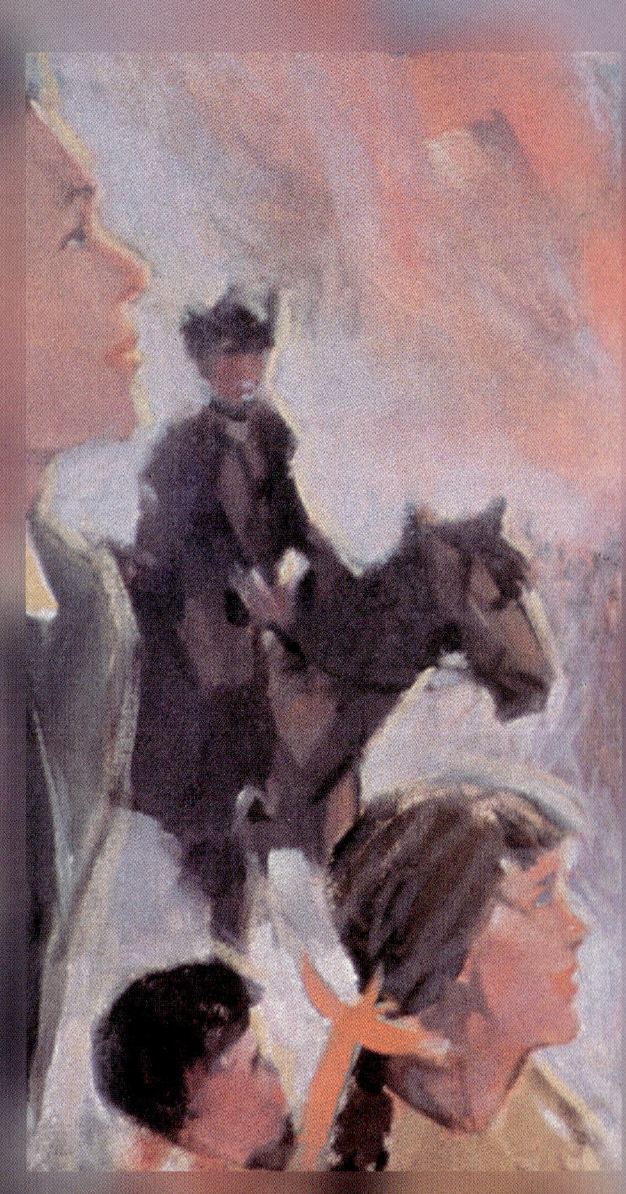

In obedience the scene is set;
the peoples and the nations are assembled.
The Lion has been made to crouch
for generations, held down in stone through
humankind's indifference and our own power
to rule by our own means. The Lord is still there
in Divine good and truth, but this is not visible to us.
"Who shall rouse Him up?" but those that are in
the good of love to Him, and who
are safe from the hells.

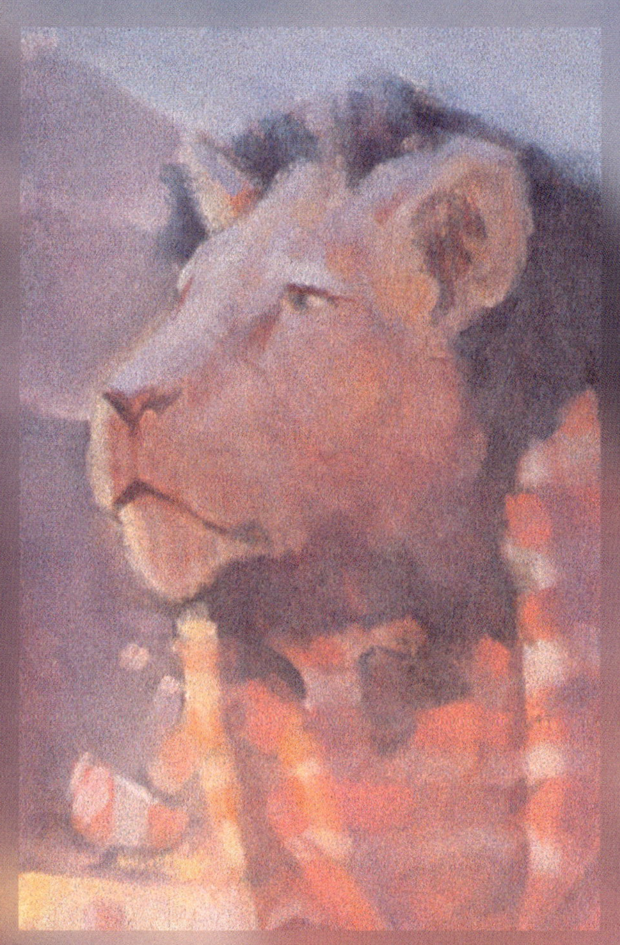

A time is at hand
for the bondage of self loves
and idolatries to be broken away,
those things which have plagued
humankind from ancient times.
The Lion begins to rise, breaking
the earthly bonds of human
minds, as a new light,
a crown, emerges
from the sky
in glory.

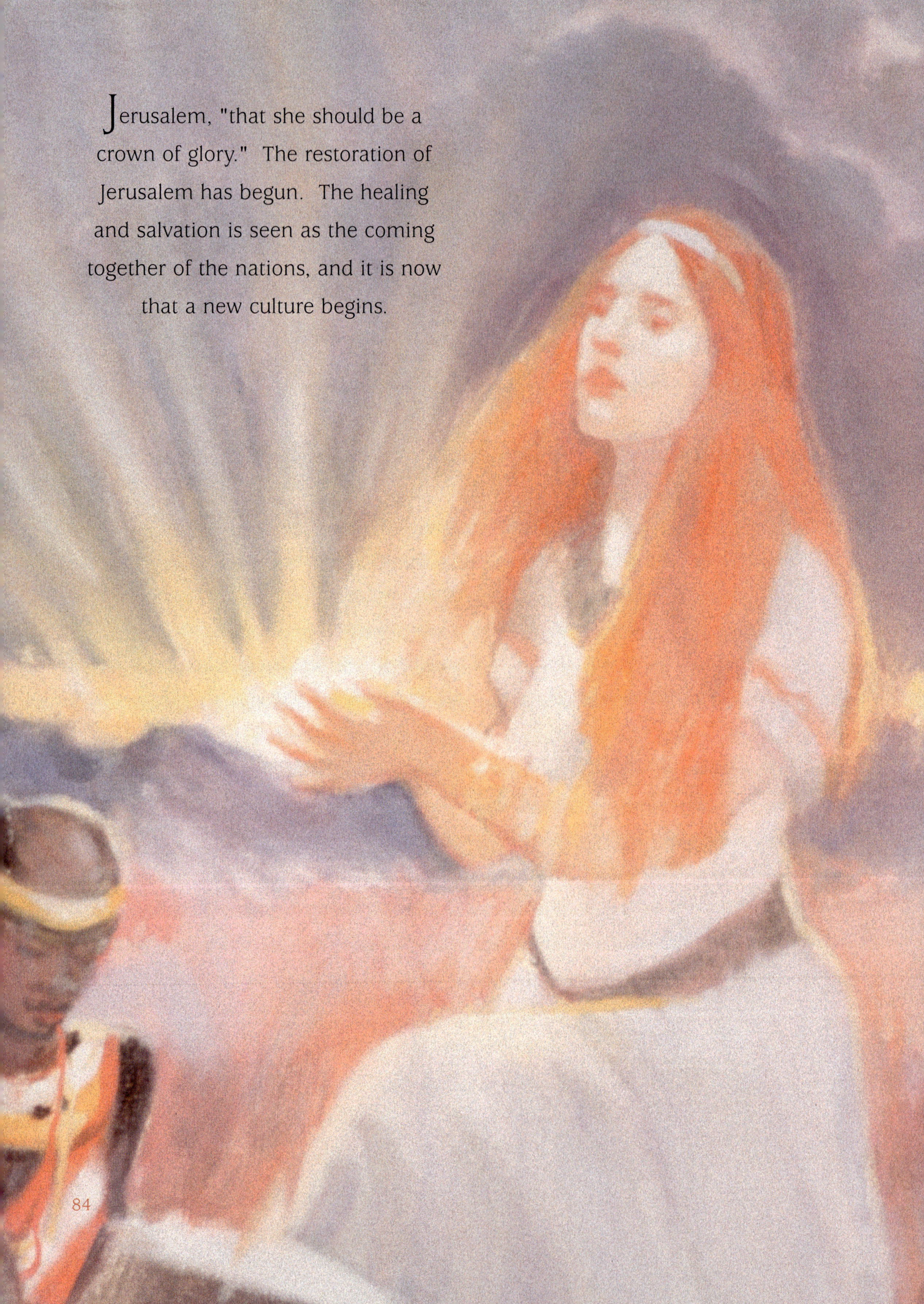

Jerusalem, "that she should be a
crown of glory." The restoration of
Jerusalem has begun. The healing
and salvation is seen as the coming
together of the nations, and it is now
that a new culture begins.

Bless the lion on the watch-tower
for His providence has guarded us,
and she who is Jerusalem shall
carry the crown of glory from the
few to the many.

Tragically a young girl died as a result of an
unfortunate car accident. I was commissioned
to do this painting with an attempt to reach
some insight through imagination. If she were
perceived in the spirit, what would she want to
say and how would she appear? Imagination is
a strange thing. It is like an ocean where both
the heavens and the earth join. To master the
imagination, one needs an idea and a willing-
ness to be led. This next painting is where
my imagination led me.

The Stars,
the Dove and the
Secret Garden

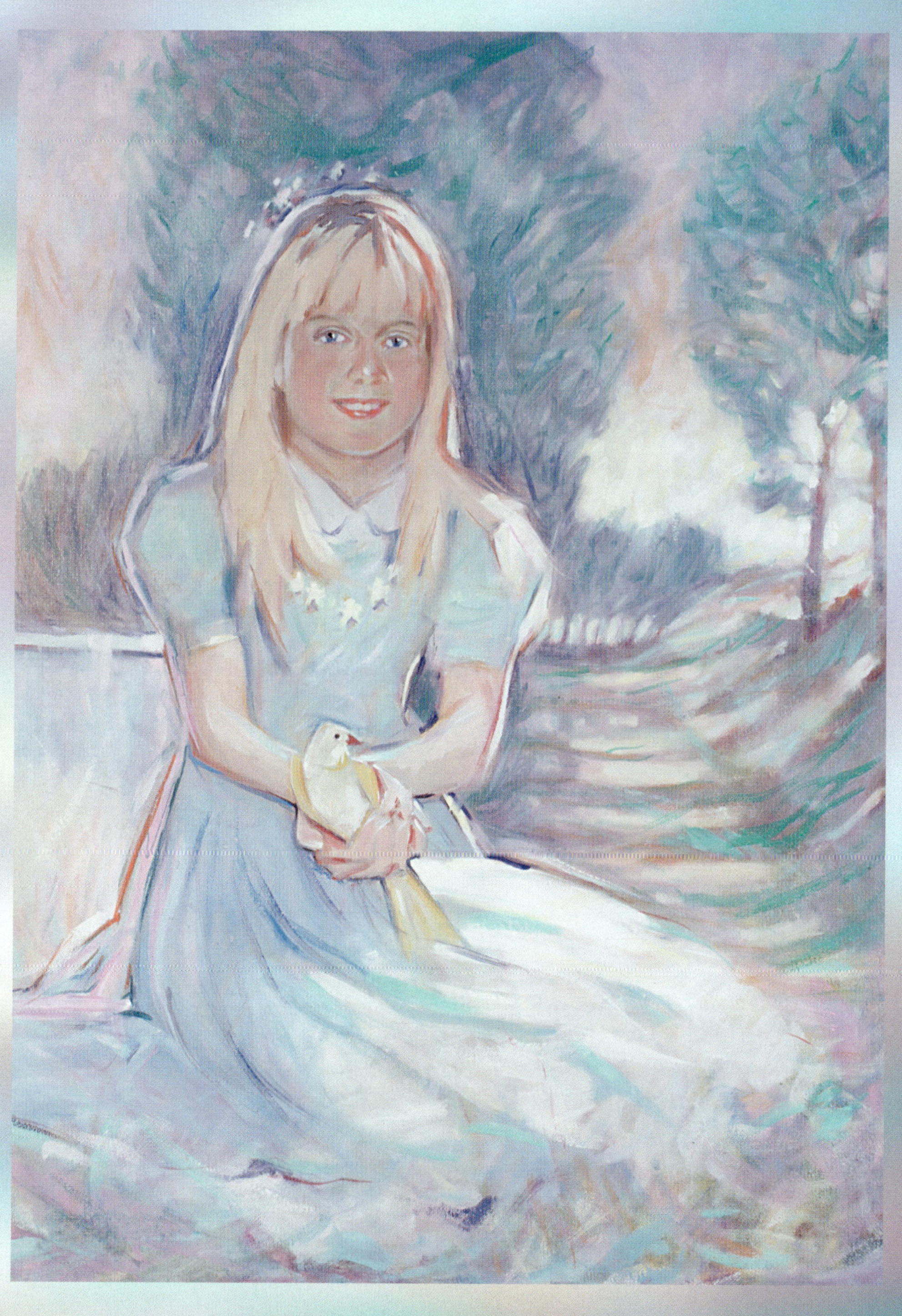

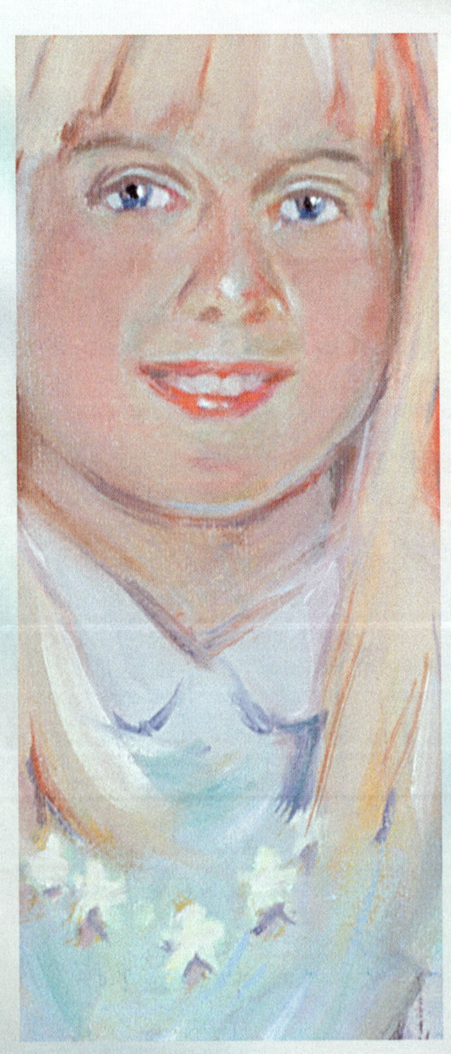

It was in a dream that I saw you.
Those eyes cannot be mistaken.
You were in a secret garden.

The stars shine,
and I hope to see a sign when I sleep,
As did the wise men long ago,
when they followed a star from the east.

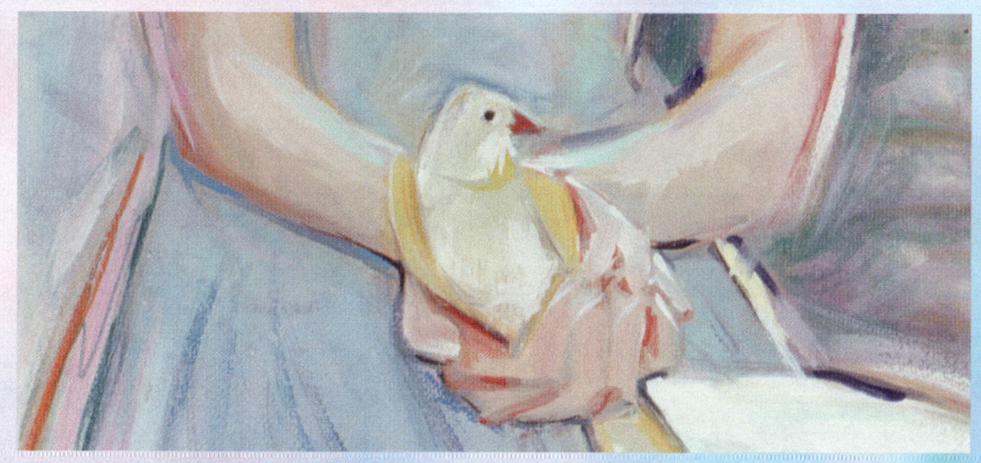

This time you hold a dove.
You knew I would be here, but the pleasure is fleeting.
Sadly the dove takes flight, and it is time for me to leave.

So until our next meeting, I will remember you,
the dove, and the secret garden.

The parable of the sower is a powerful teaching.
It talks about our reception of the Lord as He
inflows into our lives. Jesus was often most
comfortable in the company of children. Children
are receptive and are more willing to be led. It is
impossible to shield children from all the
influences of the modern world. However, it is
possible to encourage an affection for the eternal
values described through stories in the Bible.
This is the theme for this painting.

*Jesus said: Behold, a sower went forth to sow....
Some seeds fell by the wayside...some fell upon
stony places...some fell among thorns....
but other fell into good ground.*

*He that received seed into the good ground
is he that heareth the word, and understandeth it,
which also beareth fruit, and bringeth forth, some
a hundredfold, some sixty, some thirty.*

*He who hath ears to hear, let him hear.
Matthew 13:3-8, 23, 43*

The Sower

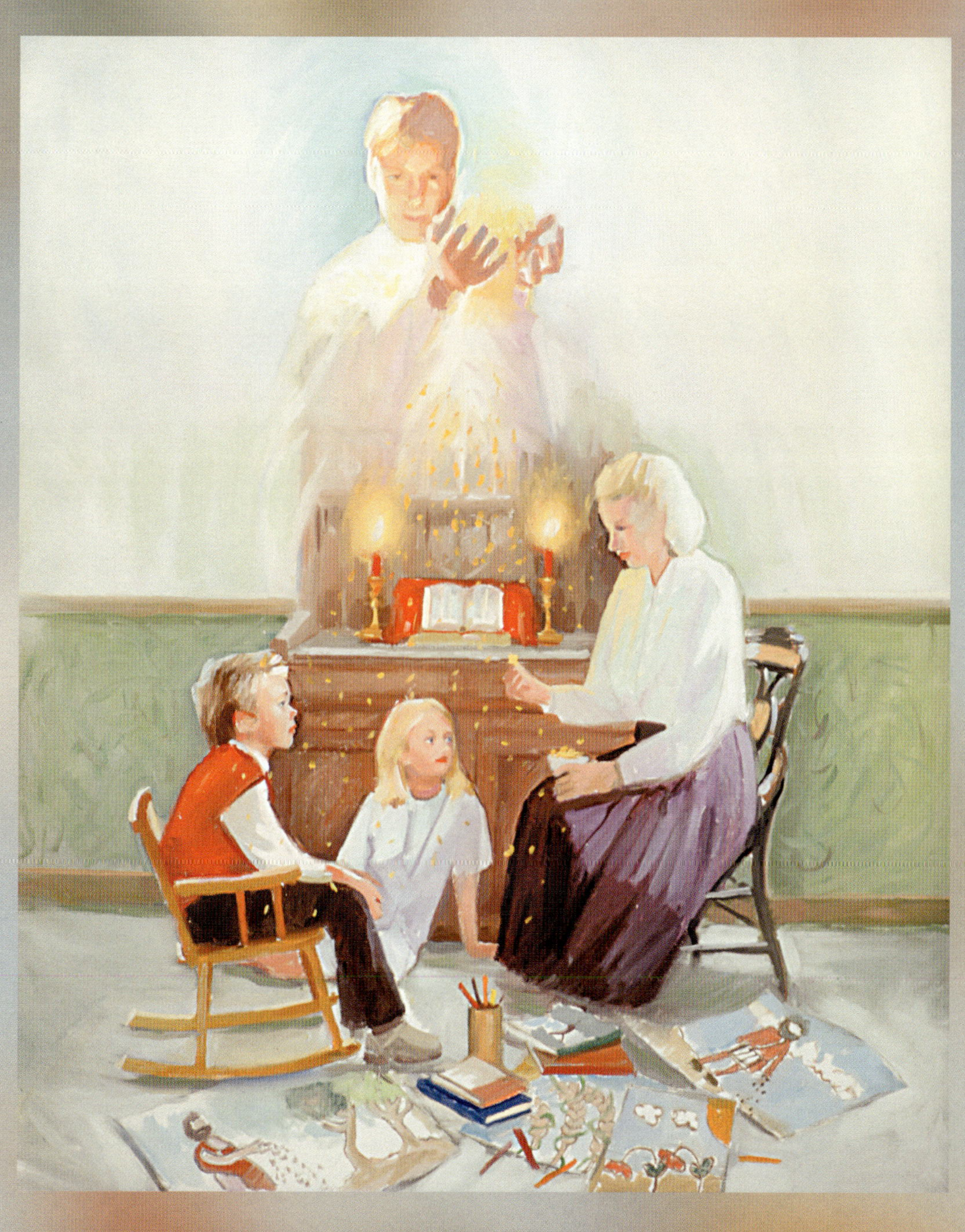

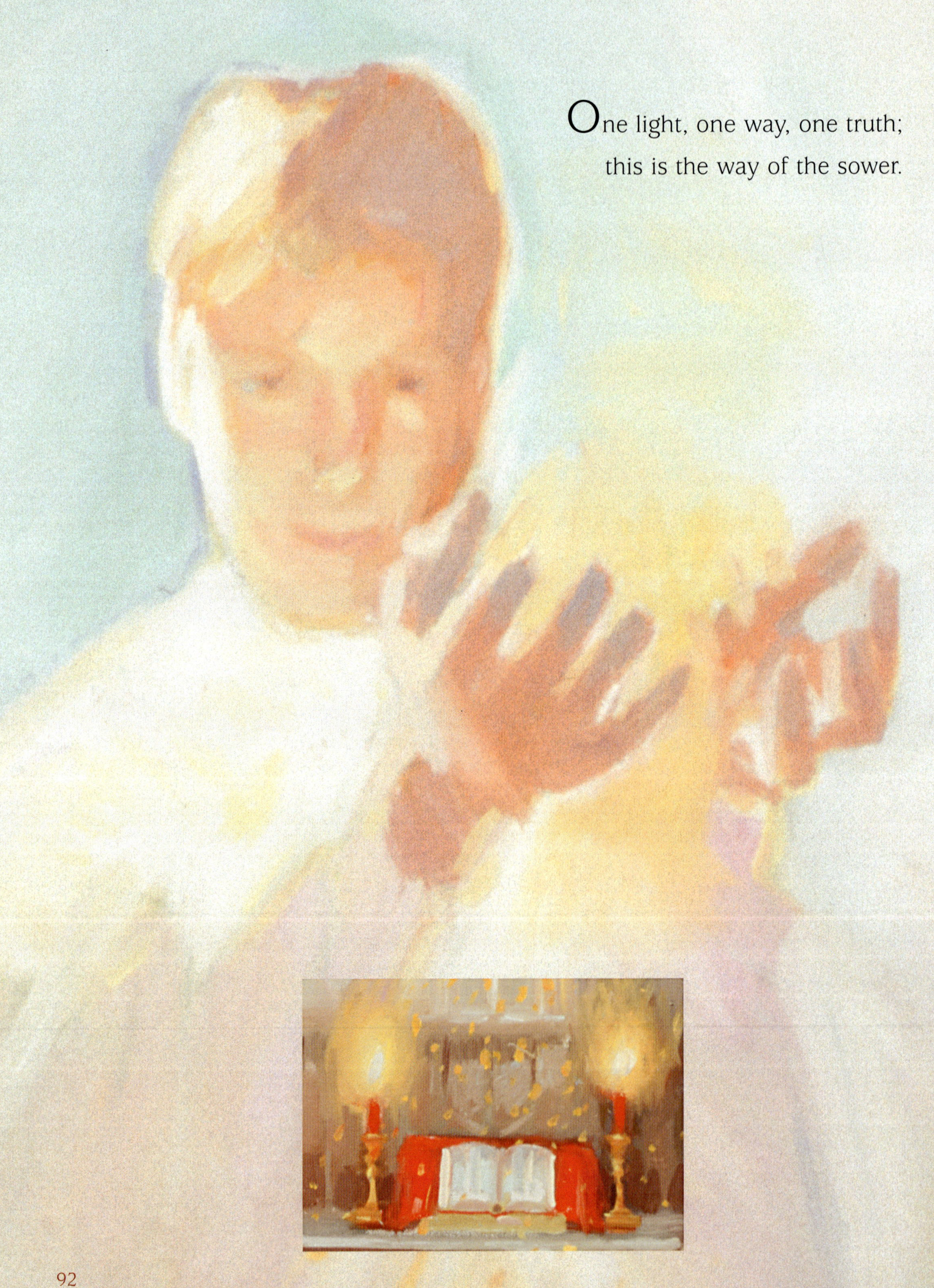

One light, one way, one truth;
this is the way of the sower.

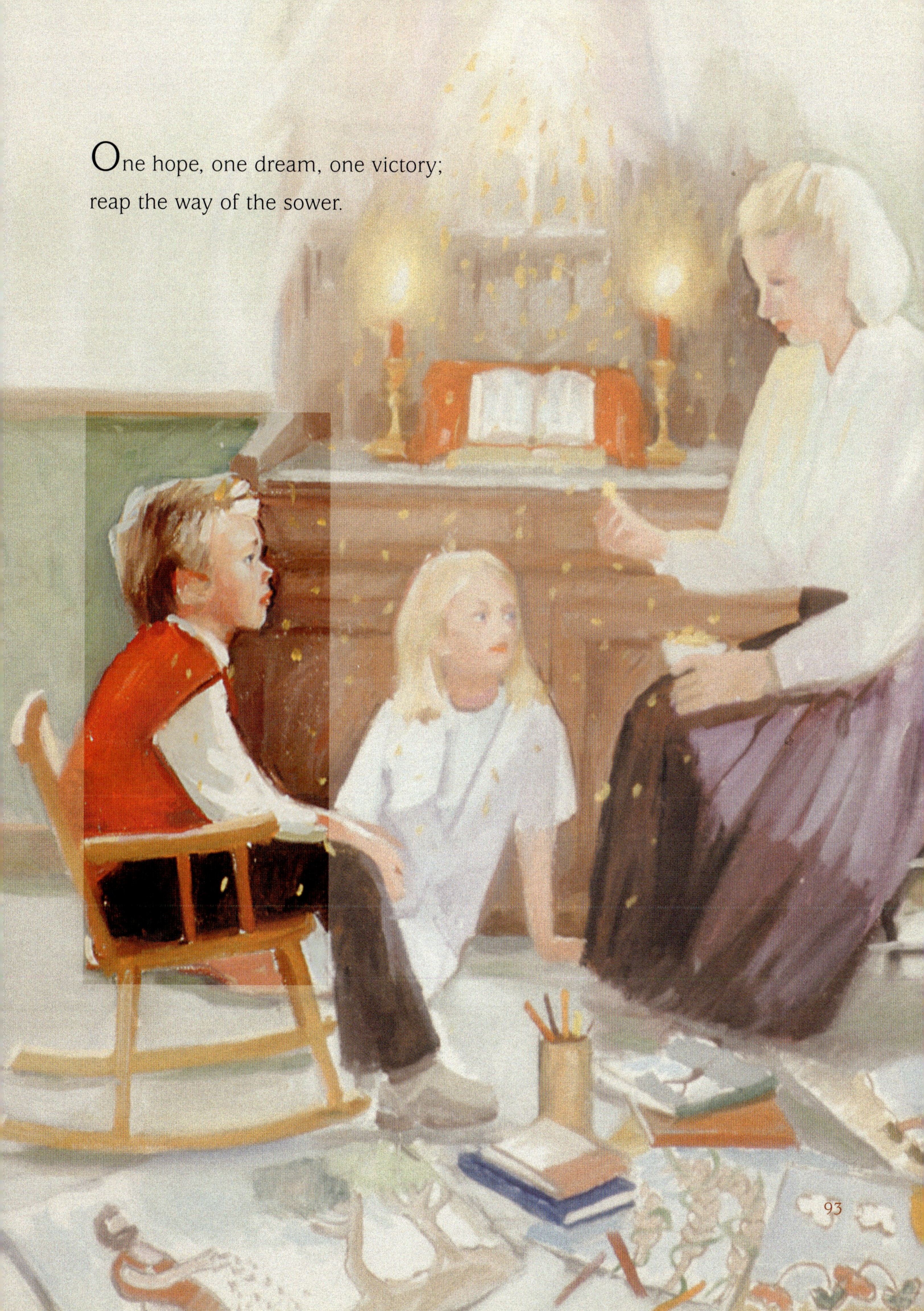

One hope, one dream, one victory;
reap the way of the sower.

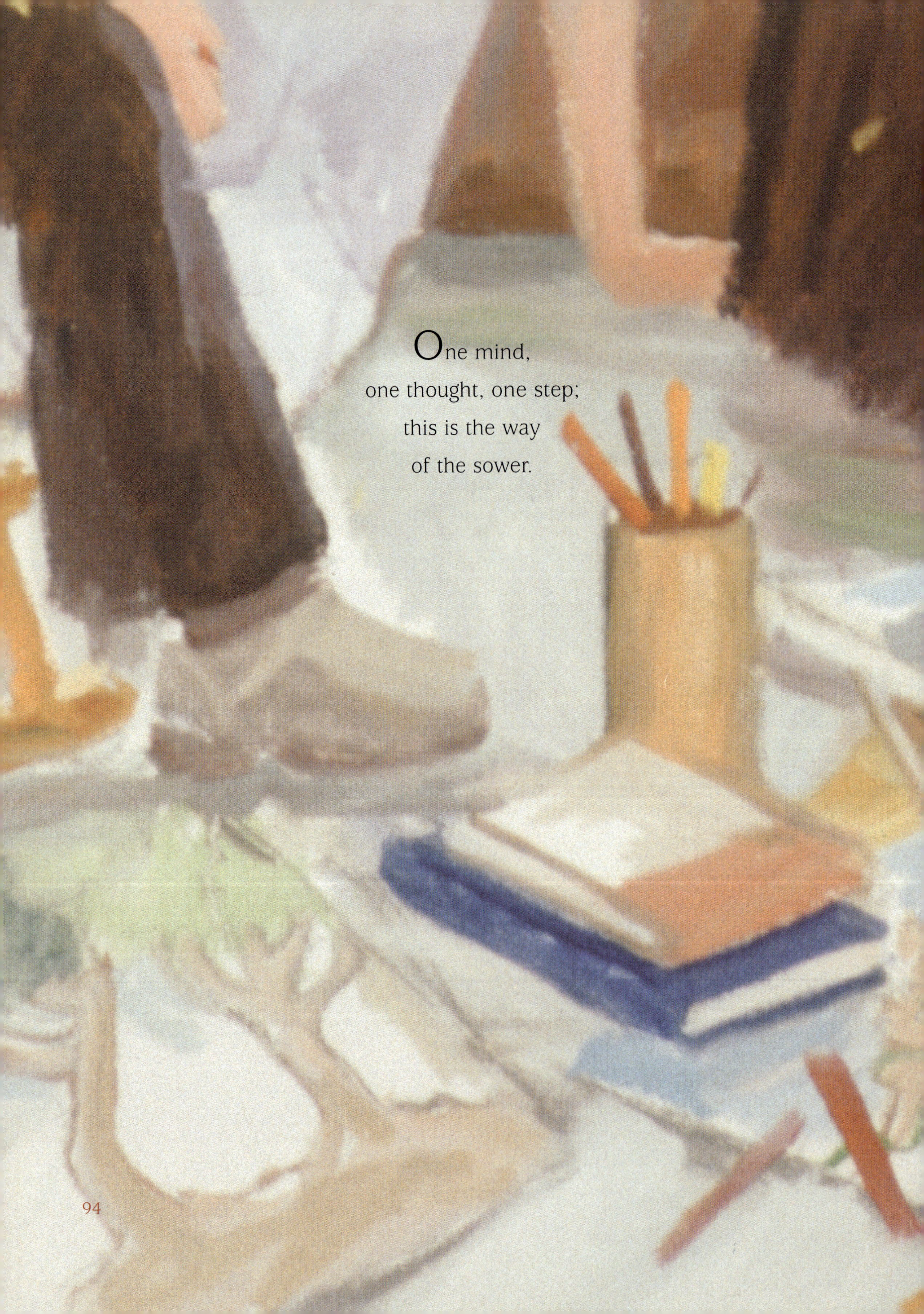

One mind,
one thought, one step;
this is the way
of the sower.

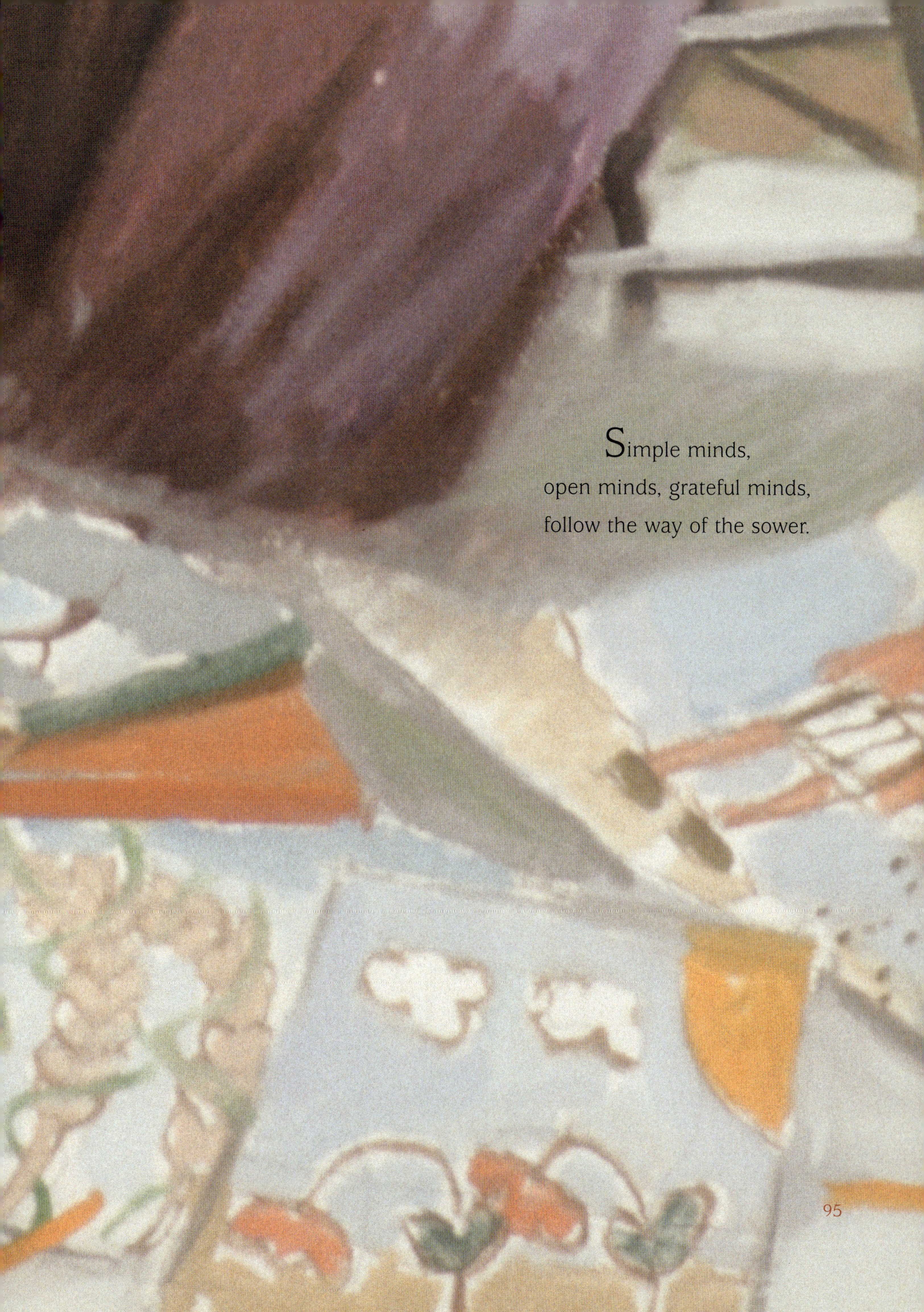
Simple minds,
open minds, grateful minds,
follow the way of the sower.

The marriage of the Lamb is come,
and his wife hath made herself ready....
Blessed are they which are called to the
marriage supper of the Lamb.
Revelation 19:7,9

I, Jesus....am the root and the offspring
of David, the bright and morning star.
And the Spirit and the bride say, Come.
And let him that heareth say, Come.
And let him that is athirst come.
Revelation 22:16,17

One of the inspirations for this painting is my daughter, Laura. I can only imagine the things she has done and the new friends she has made in the ten years since I have seen her. As a father, I know a daughter's marriage is a most special time, and one that I will not witness or experience in this world. Art and imagination serve as a bridge for me. Quotes from the Bible offer hope, and tell me that heaven is like a marriage.

Invitation
to a Wedding

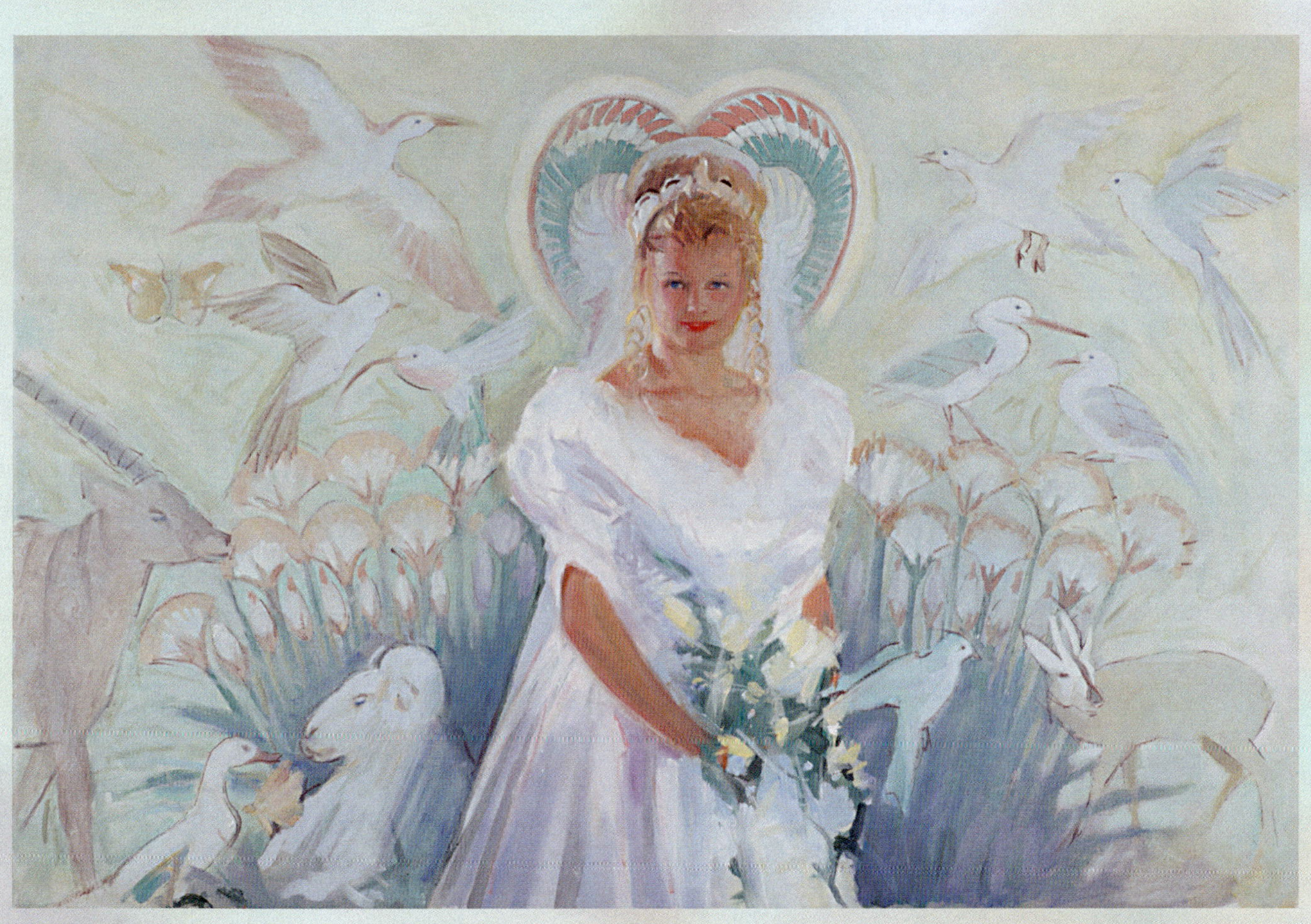

There is a woman, a bride.
"Who are you?"
To this, she just smiles.

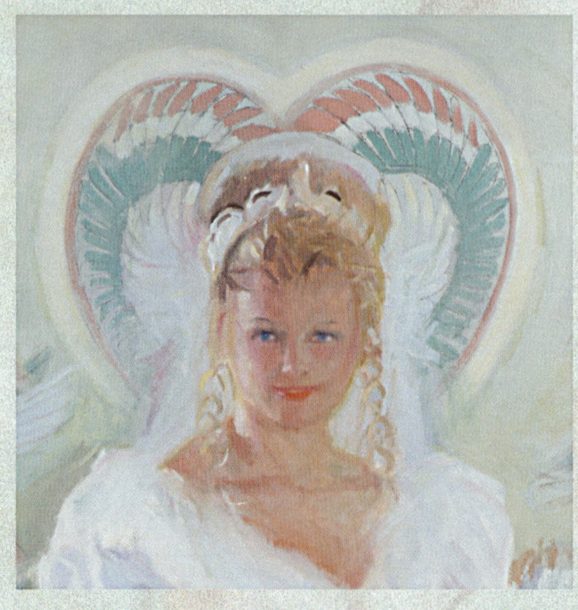

Is this a dream, or is it real?
In answer she whispers,

"The writing's on the wall."

At first I see only birds and animals.
But wait – now I see much more.
Their purpose is to tell a story.

Where you were when you were gone,
who you have become –
that is what you mean to me.

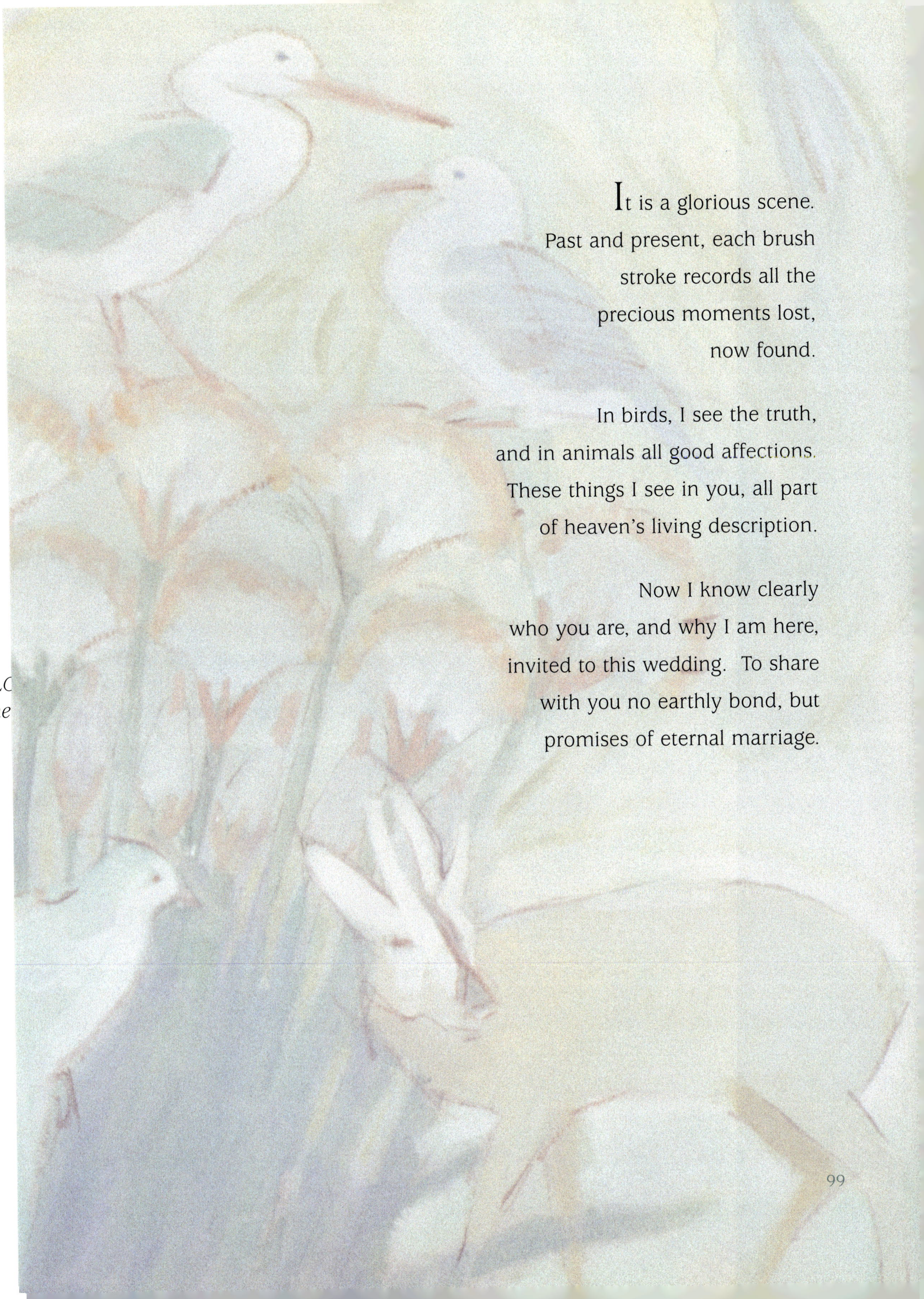

It is a glorious scene.
Past and present, each brush
stroke records all the
precious moments lost,
now found.

In birds, I see the truth,
and in animals all good affections.
These things I see in you, all part
of heaven's living description.

Now I know clearly
who you are, and why I am here,
invited to this wedding. To share
with you no earthly bond, but
promises of eternal marriage.

The LO
The

LAURA
AND
RICHARD

RYAN, DEBBIE,
JOSHUA, DANIEL
AND RICHARD

LAURA

RYAN AND LAURA

LAURA,
DEBBIE
AND
RYAN ON
RYAN'S 1ST
DAY HOME
FROM THE
HOSPITAL

LAURA

LAURA

DANIEL AND RYAN

Acknowledgments

LAURA COOK: For all the joy that she bought into my life. She taught me that happiness can shine through any obstacle. Happiness is of the spirit and obstacles are of this world. She showed me that closeness to God can be only a breath away. I thank Laura for giving me the drive to express my thoughts and feelings in art and as a result giving me the means by which I may share this with others.

EMANUEL SWEDENBORG: A special acknowledgement must be made to Emanuel Swedenborg. His theological writings have been a constant inspiration to me for many years. Without these theological writings and my resulting sound belief in an afterlife, I really do not know how I could have endured Laura's death. Through Swedenborg's revealing works I have personally experienced a perception of the spirit, and the nature of our relationship between this world and the next. Listed here are some of his books, which have provided this inspiration:
Arcana Caelestia: "When we enter a state of love or heavenly affection, we enter an angelic state." Passage #3827.
Heaven and Hell
Divine Providence
Divine Love and Wisdom
True Christian Religion: "The essence of God consists of two things, love and wisdom; while the essence of His love consists of three things, namely, to love others outside of Himself, to desire to be one with them, and from Himself to render them blessed." Passage #43

JOHN SINGER SARGENT: At the age of nine I saw his portraits. Sargent's style of painting repeatedly stood as a model for what I wished to achieve.

DAVID SHEPHERD: As a young child I saw his paintings of wildlife and steam trains which fueled my interest in art and the world around me.

NISHAN YARDUMIAN: I can easily say that this man was my first true art teacher, reaching me as a twenty-three year old student in a way that no other teacher had done before. No one has inspired or taught me as much as this man.

CEDRIC EGELI: A prominent portrait painter, who led me into developing my skills as a portrait painter.

MY WIFE DEBBIE: She is my best critic. Constantly she has provided optimism and always believed in my skills as a painter. I am greatly indebted to the detailed journals Debbie kept of Laura, which enabled me to write the first chapters of this book.

MY PARENTS: Their belief and encouragement set me on the road towards becoming an artist.

The countless friends and acquaintances that have helped shaped my confidence and my profession.

102

About the Artist

The portraiture of Richard James Cook certainly represents his winning and varied background, from receiving highest honors in art at the college level of the British school system to gaining acceptance to Cambridge College of Fine Art, and then opting to pursue a career in commercial arts. Primarily a self-taught artist, Richard went from being an Art Director to illustrator, and ultimately emerged to his final vocation as portrait painter.

Richard's portfolio is equally varied, from formal portraits such as Mr. Allen Taylor, President and C. E. O. of the Royal Bank of Canada, to the playful charm of a little girl with her Raggedy Ann.

After visiting a John Singer Sargent exhibition at the age of nine, Richard hoped to stroke the canvas with similar conviction. He had no idea then that he would be painting portraits or that he would be recognized for his achievements in portraiture. While continuing to study the great portraitists, since 1995 Richard has taken leadership from renowned portrait painter Cedric B. Egeli of Annapolis, Maryland at the Cape Cod School of Art.

Richard loves the challenge of capturing the essence of a person, especially the innocence of children. To him, portrait painting is an enriching experience and a process of getting to know his clients and subjects in a unique way.

Although based in Boston, Massachusetts, Richard accepts commissions anywhere in the United States and Canada. His portraits are in many private and corporate collections.

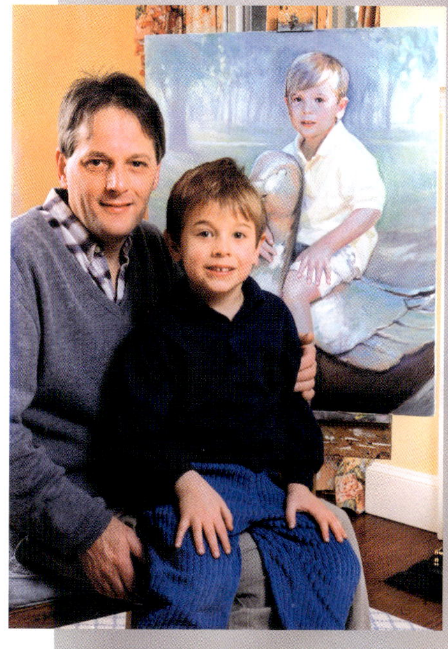

RICHARD WITH CLIENT'S SON.

SAMPLES OF RICHARD'S COMMISSIONED PORTRAITS.

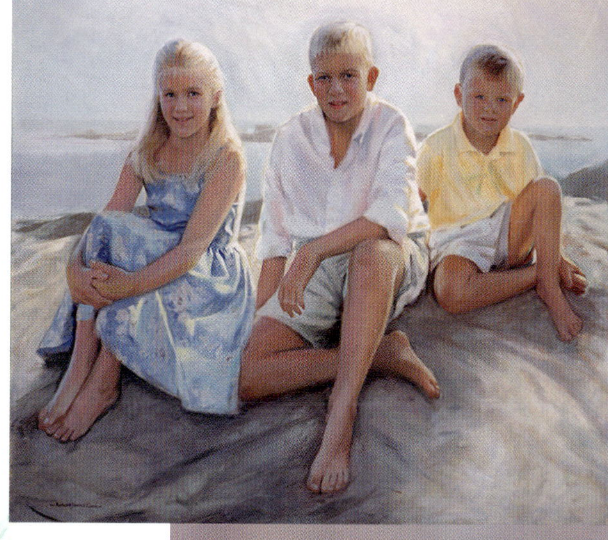

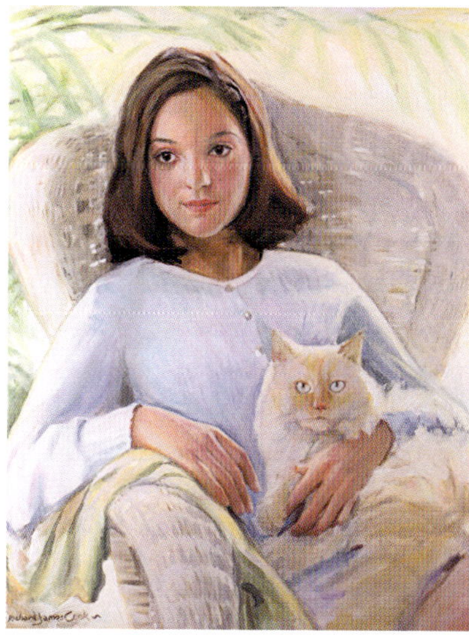

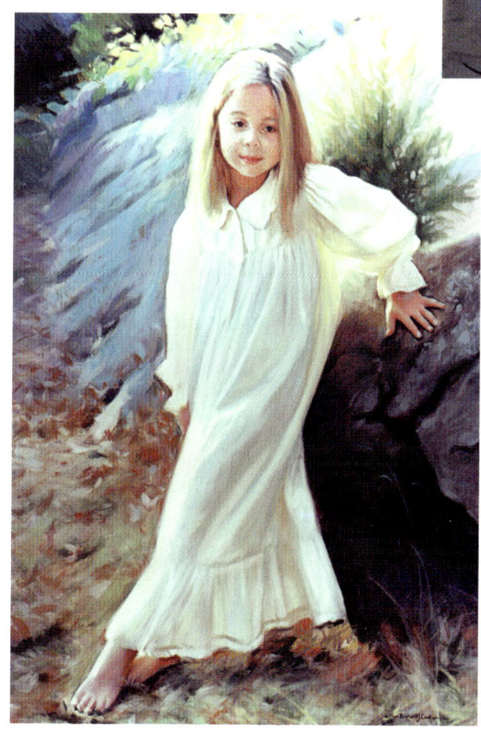

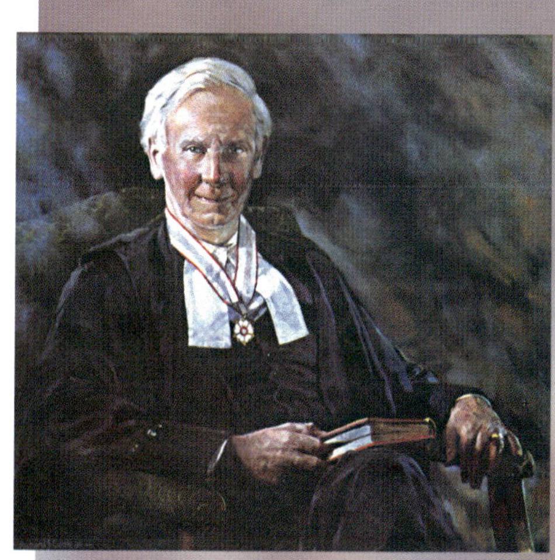

To learn more about Richard James Cook and his work, visit www.portraitartist.com/cook.

OTHER FOUNTAIN PUBLISHING TITLES YOU WILL ENJOY:

A PATH OF COLORED LEAVES - BY RACHEL CARR KLIPPENSTEIN

Rachel's story of losing the ranch that she and her husband had cherished, but then finding a challenging and exhilarating new path to follow.

"A story of starting over and acceptance; of learning from the past, and facing the future with courage. This little book holds a big message of hope, true grit and endurance." *Media Weaver—Writers NW*

"Leaves the reader feeling renewed and refreshed, ready to take on any personal dream abandoned..." *American Western –ReadtheWest.com*

"This is one of those books that makes you feel like you know the author and that they should know you." *Independent Publisher Online*

A DOVE AT THE WINDOW: LIVING DREAMS AND SPIRITUAL EXPERIENCES - EDITED BY VERA P. GLENN

True stories of comforting messages that have come from the spiritual world through dreams and visions. Each story is paired with a quotation from Swedenborg's writings.

"So many beautiful moments are included here. Each page is sure to inspire and bring a personal level of solace to the reader." *Concepts*

"[A Dove at the Window] opens new space for spiritual experiences to be shared and understood. It offers a new place to be heard." *Theta Alpha Journal*

"If anyone doubts the existence of the spiritual world, let him read *A Dove at the Window*, because it is a compelling collection." *Pittsburgh New Church Reporter*

THE WOMAN CLOTHED WITH THE SUN - INSPIRED AND ADAPTED BY BRYN J. BROCK, ILLUSTRATED BY ANNA K. COLE

The beloved story of the Woman Clothed with the Sun from the Book of Revelation, brought to life by Anna K. Cole with dramatic watercolor paintings.

"Anna Cole's bright and flowing watercolors give the woman a cosmic beauty, making her an obviously symbolic yet loving and personal figure." *New Church Life*

"Excellent watercolor paintings for children. Adults will enjoy the deep insights, based on Emanuel Swedenborg's writings, in the introduction. Vivid depiction of struggle between good and evil." *Mindquest Reviews*

"This is a book which I highly recommend to parents who wish to explore spirituality with their children." *Outlook*

THE TEMPLE OF WISDOM - BY KARIN ALFELT CHILDS

A spiritual fantasy quest adventure for readers age 10 and up, in which two young princes search for the mysterious Temple of Wisdom.

"Easy to read and exciting." *Lifeline*

"Each element of the tale receives just the right emphasis....All these things work together to create a shapely and graceful narrative." *New Church Life*

"It is rare when a book of fiction so profoundly expresses life lessons....*The Temple of Wisdom* is excellent reading for teens and young adults as well as parents of all ages." *Concepts*

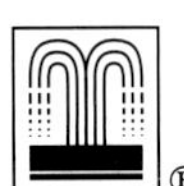

FOUNTAIN PUBLISHING®
P.O. Box 80011, Rochester, MI 48308-0011
FtnPublish@aol.com Phone: 248-651-2934
Toll-free: 877-736-8598   Fax: 248-656-4215
www.fountainpublishing.com